Treatment of Leg Veins

Procedures in Cosmetic Dermatology
Series Editor: Jeffrey S. Dover MD FRCPC
Associate Editor: Murad Alam MD

Botulinum Toxin
Alastair Carruthers MABM BCh FRCPC FRCP(Lon) and
Jean Carruthers MD FRCS(C) FRC(OPHTH)
ISBN 1 4160 2470 0

Soft Tissue Augmentation
Jean Carruthers MD FRCS(C) FRC(OPHTH) and
Alastair Carruthers MABM BCh FRCPC FRCP(Lon)
ISBN 1 4160 2469 7

Cosmeceuticals
Zoe Diana Draelos MD
ISBN 1 4160 0244 8

Laser and Lights: Volume 1
Vascular • Pigmentation • Scars • Medical Applications
David J. Goldberg MD JD
ISBN 1 4160 2386 0

Laser and Lights: Volume 2
Rejuvenation • Resurfacing • Hair Removal • Treatment of Ethnic Skin
David J. Goldberg MD JD
ISBN 1 4160 2387 9

Photodynamic Therapy
Mitchel P. Goldman MD
ISBN 1 4160 2360 7

Liposuction
C. William Hanke MD MPH FACP and Gerhard Sattler MD
ISBN 1 4160 22082

Scar Revision
Kenneth A. Arndt MD
ISBN 1 4160 31316

Chemical Peels
Mark G. Rubin MD
ISBN 1 4160 30719

Hair Transplantation
Robert S. Haber MD and Dowling B. Stough MD
ISBN 1 4160 31049

Treatment of Leg Veins
Murad Alam MD and Tri H. Nguyen MD
ISBN 1 4160 31596

Blepharoplasty
Ronald L. Moy MD and Edgar F. Fincher MD PhD
ISBN 1 4160 29966

Advanced Face Lifting
Ronald L. Moy MD and Edgar F. Fincher MD PhD
ISBN 1 4160 29974

PROCEDURES IN COSMETIC DERMATOLOGY

Series Editor: Jeffrey S. Dover MD FRCPC

Associate Editor: Murad Alam MD

Treatment of Leg Veins

Edited by

Murad Alam MD

Chief, Section of Cutaneous and Aesthetic Surgery, Departments of Dermatology and Otolaryngology-Head and Neck Surgery, Northwestern University, Chicago, IL USA

Tri H. Nguyen MD

Associate Professor, Dermatology and Otolaryngology; Director, Mohs and Dermatologic Surgery, MD Anderson Cancer Center, The University of Texas, Houston, TX, USA

Series Editor

Jeffrey S. Dover MD FRCPC

Associate Professor of Clinical Dermatology, Yale University School of Medicine, Adjunct Professor of Medicine (Dermatology), Dartmouth Medical School, Director, SkinCare Physicians of Chestnut Hill, Chestnut Hill, MA, USA

ELSEVIER
SAUNDERS

ELSEVIER
SAUNDERS

An imprint of Elsevier Inc.

© 2006, Elsevier Inc. All rights reserved.

First published 2006

ISBN-10 1 4160 31596
ISBN-13 9781416031598

British Library Cataloguing in Publication Data

A catalogue record for this book is available from the British Library

Library of Congress Cataloging in Publication Data

A catalog record for this book is available from the Library of Congress

---

Notice

Medical knowledge is constantly changing. Standard safety precautions must be followed, but as new research and clinical experience broaden our knowledge, changes in treatment and drug therapy may become necessary or appropriate. Readers are advised to check the most current product information provided by the manufacturer of each drug to be administered to verify the recommended dose, the method and duration of administration, and contraindications. It is the responsibility of the practitioner, relying on experience and knowledge of the patient, to determine dosages and the best treatment for each individual patient. Neither the Publisher nor the editor assumes any liability for any injury and/or damage to persons or property arising from this publication.

The Publisher

Printed in China

Last digit is the print number : 9 8 7 6 5 4 3 2 1

Commissioning Editor: **Karen Bowler**

Development Editors: **Martin Mellor Publishing Services Ltd, Seán Duggan, Louise Cook**

Project Managers: **Naughton Project Management, Cheryl Brant**

Illustration Manager: **Gillian Murray**

Design Manager: **Andy Chapman**

Illustrators: **Richard Prime, Tim Loughhead**

Contents

Series Foreword
Procedures in Cosmetic Dermatology

While dermatologists have been procedurally inclined since the beginning of the specialty, particularly rapid change has occurred in the past quarter century. The advent of frozen section technique and the golden age of Mohs skin cancer surgery has led to the formal incorporation of surgery within the dermatology curriculum. More recently technological breakthroughs in minimally invasive procedural dermatology have offered an aging population new options for improving the appearance of damaged skin.

Procedures for rejuvenating the skin and adjacent regions are actively sought by our patients. Significantly, dermatologists have pioneered devices, technologies and medications, which have continued to evolve at a startling pace. Numerous major advances, including virtually all cutaneous lasers and light-source based procedures, botulinum exotoxin, soft-tissue augmentation, dilute anesthesia liposuction, leg vein treatments, chemical peels, and hair transplants, have been invented, or developed and enhanced by dermatologists. Dermatologists understand procedures, and we have special insight into the structure, function, and working of skin. Cosmetic dermatologists have made rejuvenation accessible to risk-averse patients by emphasizing safety and reducing operative trauma. No specialty is better positioned than dermatology to lead the field of cutaneous surgery while meeting patient needs.

As dermatology grows as a specialty, an ever-increasing proportion of dermatologists will become proficient in the delivery of different procedures. Not all dermatologists will perform all procedures, and some will perform very few, but even the less procedurally directed amongst us must be well-versed in the details to be able to guide and educate our patients. Whether you are a skilled dermatologic surgeon interested in further expanding your surgical repertoire, a complete surgical novice wishing to learn a few simple procedures, or somewhere in between, this book and this series is for you.

The volume you are holding is one of a series entitled "Procedures in Cosmetic Dermatology." The purpose of each book is to serve as a practical primer on a major topic area in procedural dermatology.

If you want to make sure you find the right book for your needs, you may wish to know what this book is and what it is not. It is not a comprehensive text grounded in theoretical underpinnings. It is not exhaustively referenced. It is not designed to be a completely unbiased review of the world's literature on the subject. At the same time, it is not an overview of cosmetic procedures that describes these in generalities without providing enough specific information to actually permit someone to perform the procedures. And importantly, it is not so heavy that it can serve as a doorstop or a shelf filler.

What this book and this series offer is a step-by-step, practical guide to performing cutaneous surgical procedures. Each volume in the series has been edited by a known authority in that subfield. Each editor has recruited other equally practical-minded, technically skilled, hands-on clinicians to write the constituent chapters. Most chapters have two authors to ensure that different approaches and a broad range of opinions are incorporated. On the other hand, the two authors and the editors also collectively provide a consistency of tone. A uniform template has been used within each chapter so that the reader will be easily able to navigate all the books in the series. Within every chapter, the authors succinctly tell it like they do it. The emphasis is on therapeutic technique; treatment methods are discussed with an eye to appropriate indications, adverse events, and unusual cases. Finally, this book is short and can be read in its entirety on a long plane ride. We believe that brevity paradoxically results in greater information transfer because cover-to-cover mastery is practicable.

Most of the books in the series are accompanied by a high-quality DVD, demonstrating the procedures discussed in that text. Some of you will turn immediately to the DVD and use the text as a backup to clarify complex points, while others will prefer to read first and then view the DVD to see the steps in action. Choose what suits you best.

We hope you enjoy this book and the rest of the books in the series and that you benefit from the many hours of clinical wisdom that have been distilled to produce it. Please keep it nearby, where you can reach for it when you need it.

Jeffrey S. Dover MD, FRCPC and Murad Alam MD

To the women in my life

My grandmothers, Bertha and Lillian
My mother, Nina
My daughters, Sophie and Isabel
And especially to my wife, Tania

For their never-ending encouragement, patience, support, love, and friendship

To my father, Mark
A great teacher and role model

To my mentor, Kenneth A. Arndt for his generosity, kindness, sense of humor, joie de vivre, and above all else curiosity and enthusiasm

At Elsevier, Sue Hodgson who conceptualized the series and brought it to reality

and

Martin Mellor for polite, persistent, and dogged determination

Jeffrey S. Dover

The professionalism of the dedicated editorial staff at Elsevier has made this ambitious project possible. Guided by the creative vision of Sue Hodgson, Seán Duggan and Martin Mellor have attended to the myriad tasks required to produce a state-of-the-art resource. In this, they have been ably supported by the graphics team, which has maintained production quality while ensuring portability. We are also deeply grateful to the volume editors, who have generously found time in their schedules, cheerfully accepted our guidelines, and recruited the most knowledgeable chapter authors. Finally, we thank the chapter contributors, without whose work there would be no books at all. Whatever successes are herein are due to the efforts of the above, and of my teachers, Kenneth Arndt, Jeffrey Dover, Michael Kaminer, Leonard Goldberg, and David Bickers, and of my parents, Rahat and Rehana Alam.

Murad Alam

Preface

In recent years, cosmetic dermatologists have focused their efforts on reduction of the visible signs of facial aging. Aging, however, also afflicts the other end of the body: the legs and their superficial and deep vasculature. Fine red-purple telangiectasia, blue reticular veins, and bulging varicose veins lead to self-consciousness and even misery among those who feel younger than their legs look. Like facial stigmata, ugly, dysfunctional, painful legs can motivate patients to reduce their social interactions, change their dress, and compulsively frequent the cosmeceutical aisle at their neighborhood drugstore.

Leg veins are peculiar creatures. Some patients find them acutely bothersome and others do not. Similarly, some physicians find treating leg veins very rewarding, and others would rather do most any other procedure. Often, a physician's reluctance to treat leg veins derives from an uncertainty about how to proceed. Sclerotherapy of small telangiectasia is taught in many residencies, but treatment of larger vessels is less widely understood. Correction of complex leg vein disease presupposes an appreciation of the connections between the superficial and deep venous system, and a detailed knowledge of the relevant clinical anatomy of the leg.

Diagnostic methods such as Doppler and duplex ultrasound, rare tools in the dermatologist's armamentarium, are routine preliminary tests for leg vein assessment.

Indeed, effective treatment of leg veins is not always simple. Significant improvement can require multiple modalities, often delivered in a sequential or iterative manner. But while eliminating diseased leg veins requires specialized diagnostics and therapeutics, treatment success is often profoundly satisfying for the patient, and hence the physician.

The purpose of this volume is to provide clinical instruction regarding the treatment of leg veins. Sufficient clinical detail is delivered in a brief format by emphasizing practical information of direct use to the practitioner. Background material on clinical examination, diagnostic methods, instrumentation, and functional anatomy may seem dry, but comprises the necessary foundation for skillful intervention in this area.

We thank our expert contributors, many of whom are pioneers in leg vein treatment. We hope you, the reader, enjoy this book.

Murad Alam MD and Tri Nguyen MD

List of Contributors

John J. Bergan MD, FACS, FRCS, Hon(Eng), FACPh
Medical Director, Vein Institute of La Jolla; Department of Surgery, University of California, San Diego, CA, USA

Melissa A. Bogle MD
Director, Laser and Cosmetic Surgery Center of Houston, TX, USA

Joseph A. Caprini MD, MS, FACS, RVT
Louis W. Blegler Professor of Surgery and Bioengineering, Department of Surgery, Evanston Northwestern Healthcare, Evanston, IL; Professor of Biomedical Engineering, Robert R. McCormick School of Engineering and Applied Sciences, Evanston, IL; Professor of Surgery, Northwestern University Feinberg School of Medicine, Chicago, IL, USA

David M. Duffy MD
Clinical Professor of Medicine, Department of Dermatology, University of Southern California (USC), Torrance; Assistant Clinical Professor of Medicine, Department of Dermatology, University of California, Los Angeles, CA, USA

Jeffrey T.S. Hsu MD
Director of Vein Treatment Center, SkinCare Physicians of Chestnut Hill, Chestnut Hill, MA; Assistant Professor of Medicine, Department of Dermatology, Dartmouth Medical School, Hanover, NH, USA

Girish S. Munavalli MD, MHS
Medical Director, Private Practice, Goslen Aesthetic and Skin Care Center, Charlotte, NC; Clinical Instructor of Dermatology, Johns Hopkins University School of Medicine; University of Maryland-Baltimore School of Medicine, Baltimore, MD, USA

Andreas Oesch MD
Specialist for Surgery, Vein Surgery, Hirslanden Clinic, Berne, Switzerland

Luigi Pascarella MD
Postdoctorate Researcher, Department of Bioengineering, University of California, San Diego, CA, USA

Albert-Adrien Ramelet MD
Private Practice, Lausanne, Switzerland

Neil S. Sadick MD, FACP, FAACS
Clinical Professor of Dermatology, Department of Dermatology, Weill Medical College of Cornell University, New York, NY, USA

Joseph R. Schneider MD, PhD
Senior Attending, Department of Surgery, Evanston Northwestern Healthcare, Evanston; Professor, Division of Vascular Surgery, Northwestern University Medical School, Chicago, IL, USA

Robert A. Weiss MD
Director, Private Practice, Maryland Laser, Skin and Vein Institute, Hunt Valley; Associate Professor, Department of Dermatology, Johns Hopkins University School of Medicine, Baltimore, MD, USA

Steven E. Zimmet MD, FACPh
Director, Private Practice, Zimmet Vein and Dermatology Clinic, Austin, TX, USA

1 Venous Anatomy, Physiology, and Pathophysiology

John J. Bergan, Luigi Pascarella

Introduction

In order to understand treatment of various venous disorders, it is necessary to know the normal anatomy and function of the venous system of the lower extremities so as to better understand deviations from normality.

Nomenclature is particularly important since it is difficult to discuss the topic of leg veins without agreement about definitions and meaning. In 2001, an International Interdisciplinary Committee was designated by the Presidents of the International Union of Phlebology (IUP) and the International Federation of Anatomical Associations to update the official Terminologia Anatomica regarding the veins of the lower limbs. Deficiencies in the previous official Terminologia Anatomica had resulted in nonuniform anatomical nomenclature in the clinical literature that complicated international exchange of information and possibly resulted in inappropriate treatment of venous disease. The Committee, with the participation of Members of the Federative International Committee for Anatomical Nomenclature (FICAT), developed a Consensus Document at a meeting held in Rome on the occasion of the 14th World Congress of the IUP. Recommendations of the Committee were published and these new, occasionally unfamiliar terms are used in the following exposition.

Anatomy

The venous system in the lower extremities can be divided, for purposes of understanding, into three systems: the deep system, which parallels the tibia and femur; the superficial venous system, which resides in the superficial tissue compartment between the deep muscular fascia and the skin; and the perforating or connecting veins, which join the superficial to the deep systems. The perforating veins are thus named because they penetrate anatomical barriers.

Although the superficial veins are the targets of most therapies, the primary return of blood flow from the lower extremities is through the deep veins. In the calf, these deep veins are paired with and named for their accompanying arteries. Specifically, the anterior tibial, posterior tibial, and peroneal arteries are accompanied by their paired veins, to which they are interconnected. These crural veins join to form the popliteal vein. Occasionally the popliteal vein and femoral vein are paired.

As the popliteal vein ascends, it becomes the femoral vein, formerly called the superficial femoral vein. Near the groin, the femoral vein joins the deep femoral vein, and the two become the common femoral vein, which ascends to become the external iliac vein proximal to the inguinal ligament.

Ultrasound imaging has shown that the superficial compartment of the lower extremity is in fact comprised of two compartments, one enclosing all of the structures between the muscular fascia and the skin. The other is within the superficial compartment and encloses the saphenous vein. It is bounded by the muscular fascia inferiorly and the superficial fascia superiorly. It is termed the 'saphenous compartment' (Fig. 1.1). The importance of this anatomic structure, the saphenous compartment, is underscored by its being targeted during percutaneous placement of endovenous catheters and the instillation of tumescent anesthesia.

The main superficial veins are the great saphenous vein (GSV) and small saphenous vein. Each of these has many interconnecting tributaries, referred to as communicating veins. The GSV originates on the dorsum of the foot, from where it ascends anterior to the medial malleolus of the ankle and further onto the anteromedial aspect of the tibia. At the knee, the GSV is found in the medial aspect of the popliteal space. It then ascends through the anteromedial thigh to join the common femoral vein just below the inguinal ligament. Throughout its course, it lies within the saphenous compartment. The

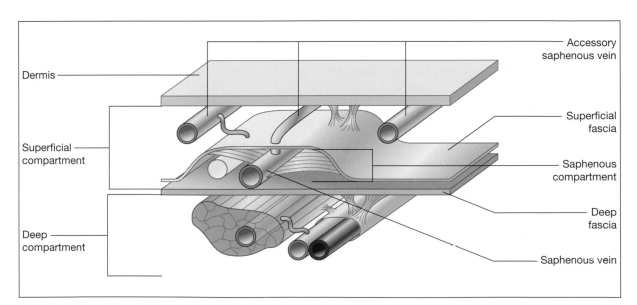

Fig. 1.1 This diagram of the saphenous compartment shows its relationships with the superficial and deep compartments as well as the saphenous vein (SV) and nerve and their relationships to the medial, anterior and lateral accessory saphenous veins (ASVs). (Redrawn from Caggiati A, Bergan JJ, Gloviczki P, Jantet G, Wendell-Smith CP, Partsch H 2002 International Interdisciplinary Consensus Committee on Venous Anatomical Terminology. Nomenclature of the veins of the lower limbs: an international interdisciplinary consensus statement. Journal of Vascular Surgery 36:416–422)

small saphenous vein originates laterally from the dorsal venous arch of the foot and travels subcutaneously behind the lateral malleolus at the ankle. As it ascends in the calf, it enters the deep fascia and courses between the heads of the gastrocnemius muscle to join the popliteal vein behind the knee (Fig. 1.2). Significantly, there are many anatomic

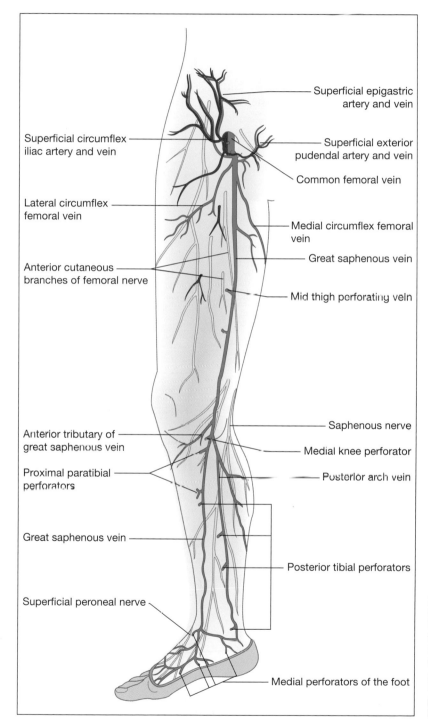

Superficial epigastric artery and vein

Superficial circumflex iliac artery and vein

Superficial exterior pudendal artery and vein

Common femoral vein

Lateral circumflex femoral vein

Medial circumflex femoral vein

Great saphenous vein

Anterior cutaneous branches of femoral nerve

Mid thigh perforating vein

Saphenous nerve

Anterior tributary of great saphenous vein

Medial knee perforator

Proximal paratibial perforators

Posterior arch vein

Great saphenous vein

Posterior tibial perforators

Superficial peroneal nerve

Medial perforators of the foot

Fig. 1.2 This diagrammatic representation of the GSV emphasizes it relationship to perforating veins and the posterior arch vein. (Redrawn from Mózes G, Gloviczki P, Kádár A, Carmichael SW 1998 Anatomy of the perforating veins in Gloviczki P and Bergan JJ (eds) Atlas of endoscopic perforating vein surgery. Springer, London

variations in the orientation of the small saphenous vein regarding its points of connection to the popliteal vein, cranial extensions of the saphenous vein, and posteromedial circumflex vein (vein of Giacomini).

The third system of veins, the perforating vein system, connects the superficial and deep systems of veins. The direction of fluid flow within the perforating veins may not be intuitively clear. Some perforating veins produce normal flow from the superficial to the deep circulation while others conduct abnormal outflow from the deep circulation to the superficial circulation, so-called perforating vein reflux. Indeed, any of the perforating veins may develop bi-directional flow (Table 1.1; Fig. 1.3).

These medial perforating veins may become targets for treatment of severe chronic venous insufficiency. Smaller perforating veins found along the intermuscular septa allow direct drainage of blood from surface veins into the deep venous system. Conversely, when they are dysfunctional, these small perforators allow muscular compartment pressure to be transmitted directly to cutaneous and subcutaneous veins and venules.

Venous Physiology

It is estimated that 60–75% of the blood in the body is found in the veins. Of this, about 80% is contained in veins that are smaller than

Summary of important changes in nomenclature of lower extremity veins	
Old terminology	**New terminology**
Femoral vein	Common femoral vein
Superficial femoral vein	Femoral vein
Sural veins	Sural veins
Soleal veins	
Gastrocnemius veins (Medial and lateral)	
Huntarian perforator	Mid-thigh perforator
Cockett's perforators	Paratibial perforator
Posterior tibial perforators	
May's perforator	
Gastrocnemius point	Intergemellar perforator

Table 1.1 Summary of important changes in nomenclature of lower extremity veins

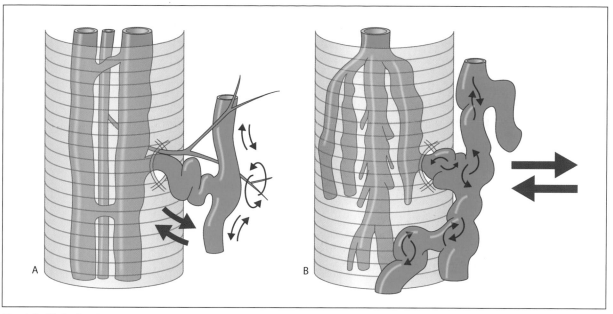

Fig. 1.3 (**A**) Perforating vein connecting an incompetent superficial vein to the tibial circulation. This is a reentry perforator elongated and dilated by increased volume flow. (**B**) Incompetent outflow or exit perforator causing elongation and dilation of superficial veins

200 μm in diameter. Thus the small veins function as a reservoir for much of the body's blood volume. Further, the splanchnic venous circulation and cutaneous veins are richly supplied by the sympathetic nervous system fibers while muscular veins are innervated with few or none of these. The veins in skeletal muscle, on the other hand, are responsive to catecholamines.

Although arterial pressures are generated by muscular contractions of the heart, pressures in the venous system are largely determined by gravity. With the body in the horizontal position, pressures in the veins of the lower extremity are similar to the pressures in the abdomen, chest, and extended arm. However, movement to an upright position results in dramatic changes in venous pressure. The only point in which the pressure remains constant is a stable point just below the diaphragm. All pressures distal to this point are increased due to the weight of the blood column from the right atrium. In the upright position, largely due to reflux through the valveless vena cava and iliac veins, there is an accumulation of approximately 500 ml of blood in the lower extremities. Some of this fluid diffuses into the tissues, is collected by the lymphatic system, and eventually returns to the venous system.

Venous valves play an important role in transporting blood from the lower extremities to the heart. Upward movement is contingent on valve closure, and in order for valve closure to occur, there must be a reversal of the normal transvalvular pressure gradient. Back pressure resulting in flow exceeding 30 cm/second leads to valve closure

(Fig. 1.4). Direct observation of human venous valves via specialized ultrasound techniques has revealed that venous flow is normally not in a steady state but is pulsatile. Venous valves undergo regular opening and closing cycles. Even when fully opened, the cross-sectional area between the leaflets is 35% smaller than that of the vein distal to the valve. Flow through the valve separates into a proximally directed jet and distal flow into the sinus pocket proximal to the valve cusp. The vortical flow prevents statis and ensures that all surfaces of the valve are exposed to shear stress. Valve closure develops when the vortical flow pressure exceeds the proximally directed jet flow.

Intuitively, the role of venous valves during muscular exercise is to promote antegrade flow from superficial veins to deep veins while preventing retrograde motion in the opposite direction. Normally functioning perforating vein valves protect the skin and subcutaneous tissues from the effects of muscular contraction pressure, possibly exceeding 100–130 mmHg, which may cause pooling of fluid in the superficial circulation. In particular, volume and pressure changes in

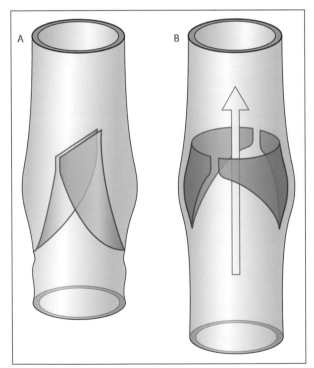

Fig. 1.4 Venous valves are crucial to blood flow from the lower extremities to the heart. Proximal movement is contingent on valve closure (**A**). In order for valve closure to occur, there must be a reversal of the normal transvalvular pressure gradient. Back pressure resulting in flow exceeding 30 cm/second leads to valve closure. (**B**) Valve leaflets are shown fully opened, allowing upward flow. Redrawn from Tibbs DJ 1992 Varicose veins and related disorders. Butterworth Heinemann, London

veins within the calf occur with muscular activity. In the resting position, with the foot flat on the floor, there is no muscle-instigated flow. However, in the heel strike position, the venous plexus under the heel and plantar surface of the foot (Bejar's plexus) is emptied proximally. Properly functioning valves ensure that blood flows from the foot and ankle into the deep veins of the calf. Then, calf contraction transports this blood into the deep veins of the thigh, and henceforth, blood flow proceeds to the pelvic veins, vena cava, and ultimately to the heart, all due to the influence of lower extremity muscular contraction.

The role of venous valves in an individual quietly standing is not well understood. Pressures in the superficial and deep veins should theoretically be the same during quiet standing, but as Arnoldi has found, the pressure in the deep veins is 1 mm higher, which would tend to keep the valves in the perforating veins closed.

Pathophysiology

Abnormal functioning of the veins of the lower extremities is recognized clinically as venous dysfunction or, more commonly, venous insufficiency. Cutaneous telangiectasias and subcutaneous varicose veins are usually grouped under the rubric 'primary venous insufficiency' while lower limbs with hyperpigmentation, edema and healed or open venous ulceration are indicative of chronic venous insufficiency (CVI).

Primary Venous Insufficiency

Understanding of the pathophysiology of venous insufficiency has improved during the past few years. It is currently believed that a dysfunctional venous system can result from injury to vein walls and venous valves. This type of injury entails acquired severe inflammation exacerbated by other factors, such as heredity, obesity, female gender, pregnancy and a standing occupation. Vein wall injury allows the vein to elongate and dilate, thus producing an increase in vein diameter, valve dysfunction, reflux, and the visual manifestations of varicose veins. Specifically, the effect of persistent reflux through axial veins is a chronic increase in distal venous pressure. This venous pressure increases from the inguinal ligament past the knee to the ankle. Prolonged venous hypertension resulting from venous pressure initiates a cascade of pathologic events that manifest as lower extremity edema, pain, itching, skin discoloration and ulceration.

The earliest signs of venous insufficiency are often elongated and dilated veins within the epidermis and dermis. These are called telangiectasias. Slightly deeper and under the skin are flat, blue–green veins of the reticular (network) system. These may become dilated and elongated as well (Fig. 1.5). Finally, even deeper but still above the superficial fascia are the varicose veins. All of these abnormal veins and venules are similar in that they are elongated, tortuous and connected to dysfunctional venous valves.

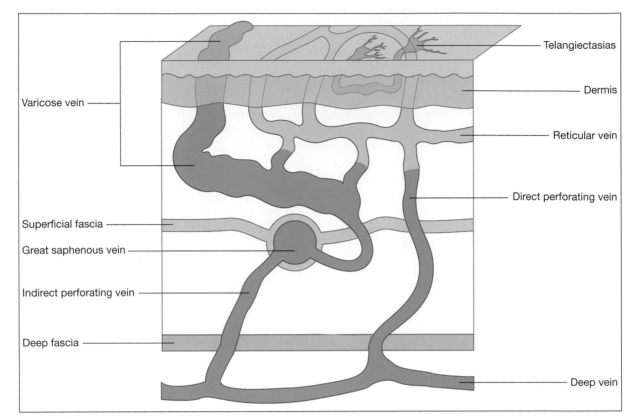

Fig. 1.5 This cross-sectional view of the subcutaneous venous circulation shows how venous hypertension is transmitted to the unsupported veins of the dermis and subcutaneous tissues from axial veins (GSV) and the deep veins of the muscular compartments. (Redrawn from Somjen GM 1995 Anatomy of the superficial venous system. Dermatologic Surgery 21:35–45)

Chronic Venous Insufficiency

Postinflammatory hyperpigmentation, scarring from previous ulceration, and active ulcerations are grouped together under the term 'chronic venous insufficiency.' Numerous incomplete and discredited theories have been postulated regarding the cause of CVI and the cause of venous ulceration. An early example is the theory of venous stasis first proposed in a manuscript by John Homans of Harvard in 1916. Dr Homans, who first coined the term 'post-phlebitic syndrome' to describe the skin changes of CVI, suggested that 'overstretching of the vein walls and destruction of the valves ... interferes with the nutrition of the skin ... therefore, skin which is bathed under pressure with stagnant venous blood will form permanent open sores or ulcers.' The erroneous term 'stasis ulcer' honors that misconception, as do the terms 'venous stasis disease' and 'stasis dermatitis.'

Alfred Blalock, a pioneer in cardiac surgery, disproved the stasis theory by studying oxygen content from varicose veins and normal veins. He observed that the oxygen content of the femoral vein in patients with severe chronic venous insufficiency was greater than the oxygen content of the contralateral nonaffected limb. This finding led some investigators to conclude that arteriovenous fistulas caused venous stasis and varicose veins. That explanation, though simplistic, has some basis in fact since the thermal regulatory apparatus in limbs depends on the opening and closing of arteriovenous shunts. The presence of these shunts explains some severe adverse events that occur during sclerotherapy, when sclerosant entering a vein is shunted into the arterial system and redistributed. However, although these shunts actually exist and do open under conditions of venous hypertension, investigations using microspheres have failed to validate the theory that arteriovenous fistulas cause varicose veins.

Hypoxia and its part in causing CVI was investigated during the last two decades of the 20th century. Investigators came to believe that a fibrin cuff, observed histologically, blocked transport of oxygen and was responsible for skin changes of CVI at the ankles and distally. That theory has been abandoned, even though a true periarteriolar cuff is easily identified histologically.

It is now suspected that the manifestations of lower extremity venous insufficiency derive from two phenomena related to venous hypertension: (1) failure of the vein valves and vein walls; and (2) skin changes at the ankles.

Failure of Vein Walls and Valves

The authors' work suggests that venous hypertension causes a shear-stress-dependent leukocyte–endothelial interaction, which is characterized by chronic inflammation. Microscopic events include leukocyte rolling, firm adhesion to endothelium, and subsequent migration of the cells through the endothelial barrier into parenchyma of valves and vein walls. There, macrophages elaborate matrix metalloproteases, which destroy elastin and possibly collagen as well. Vein walls become stretched and elongated. Vein valves become perforated, torn and even scarred to the point of near-total ablation. Changes are eventually seen both macroscopically and angioscopically. Similar changes have been produced in the animal models by constructing an arteriovenous fistula to mimic venous hypertension in man.

Skin Changes

The second manifestation of CVI is in skin changes. There is evidence that leukocyte activation in the skin, perhaps related to venous hypertension, plays a major role in the pathophysiology of CVI. Thomas, working with Dormandy, was the first to implicate abnormal leukocyte activity in this process. They reported that 25% fewer white blood cells and platelets exited the dependent foot of patients with venous hypertension when compared to normal individuals. When the foot was elevated, there was a significant washout of white blood cells but not platelets, suggesting platelet consumption within the microcirculation of the dependent foot. The investigators concluded that the decrease in white cell exodus was due to leukocyte trapping in the venous microcirculation secondary to venous hypertension. They further speculated that trapped leukocytes may become activated, resulting in release of toxic metabolites causing damage to the microcirculation and overlying skin. Apparently, the incipient injury in the skin is extravasation of red blood cell degradation products and proteins into the dermal interstitium. These released substances are potent chemoattractants that represent the initial chronic inflammatory signal responsible for leukocyte recruitment.

The importance of leukocytes in the development of dermal skin alterations has been further explored by Coleridge Smith and colleagues. After obtaining punch biopsies from patients with primary varicose veins, lipodermatosclerosis, and healed ulcers, they counted the median number of white blood cells per high-power field in each group. There was no attempt to identify the type of leukocytes. In patients with primary varicose veins, lipodermatosclerosis, and healed ulceration, there was a median of 6, 45 and 217 white blood cells per cubic millimeter, respectively. A correlation was thus established between clinical disease severity and the number of leukocytes in the dermis of patients with CVI.

It remains poorly understood which types of leukocytes are most active in venous stasis skin changes. Several types, including T-lymphocytes, macrophages and mast cells, have been observed on immunohistochemical and electron microscopic examination. Part of this variation may be explained by patient differences. Patients with more eczematous skin changes may have an autoimmune component to their CVI whereas patients with dermal fibrosis may have findings more consistent with chronic inflammation and altered tissue remodeling. Accompanying the infiltration of leukocytes into the extracellular space is disorganized collagen deposition.

Summary and Conclusion

Knowing the normal anatomy of the venous system of the lower extremities and the normal functioning of its elements is essential to understanding the pathologic processes of venous dysfunction. Valve and vein wall damage, as well as the advanced skin changes of CVI, result from sterile inflammatory reactions. Both phenomena appear to be triggered by venous hypertension and, therefore, therapy must be directed at correcting such venous hypertension.

Further reading

Arnoldi CC 1965 Venous pressures in the leg of healthy human subjects at rest and during muscular exercise in the nearly erect position. Acta Chirurgica Scandinavica 130:520–534

Ballard JL, Bergan JJ 2000 Chronic venous insufficiency: Diagnosis and treatment. Springer-Verlag, London Berlin Heidelberg

Bergan JJ, Weiss RA, Goldman MP 2000 Extensive tissue necrosis following high-concentration sclerotherapy for varicose veins. Dermatologic Surgery 26:535–542

Blalock A 1929 Oxygen content of blood in patients with varicose veins. Archives of Surgery 19:898–904

Brewer AC 1950 Arteriovenous shunts. British Medical Journal 2:270

Browse NL, Burnand KG 1998 The cause of venous ulceration. Lancet ii:243–245

Bundens WP, Bergan JJ, Halasz NA, Murray J, Drehobl M 1995 The superficial femoral vein: a potentially lethal misnomer. JAMA 274:1296–1298

Bush RG, Hammond KA 1999 Tumescent anesthetic technique for long saphenous stripping. Journal of the American College of Surgery 189:626–628

Caggiati A, Bergan JJ, Gloviczki P, Jantet G, Wendell-Smith CP, Partsch H 2002 International Interdisciplinary Consensus Committee on Venous Anatomical Terminology. Nomenclature of the veins of the lower limbs: an international interdisciplinary consensus statement. Journal of Vascular Surgery 36:416–422

Coleridge Smith PD 2001 Microcirculation disorders in venous leg ulcer. Microcirculation in CVI. Microcirculation 1–10

Federative International Committee for Anatomical Terminology 1998 Terminologia anatomica. George Thieme Verlag, Stuttgart

Gardner AMN, Fox RH 1993 The return of blood to the heart. 2nd edn. John Libbey Publisher, London, p 81

Homans J 1916 The operative treatment of varicose veins and ulcers based on a classification of these lesions. Surgical Gynecology and Obstetrics 22:143–158

Homans J 1917 The etiology and treatment of varicose ulcer of the leg. Surgical Gynecology and Obstetrics 24:300–311

Hoshino S, Satokawa H, Ono T, Igari T 1992 Surgical treatment for varicose veins of the legs using intraoperative angioscopy. In: Raymond-Martimbeau P, Prescott R, Zummo M (eds) Phlebologie 92. John Libbey Eurotext, Paris, pp 1083–1085

Lurie F, Kistner RL, Eklof B, Kessler D 2003 Mechanism of venous valve closure and role of the valve in circulation: a new concept. Journal of Vascular Surgery 38:955–961

Pappas PJ, DeFouw DO, Venezio LM, et al 1997 Morphometric assessment of the dermal microcirculation in patients with chronic venous insufficiency. Journal of Vascular Surgery 26:784–795

Piulachs P, Vidal Baraquer F 1953 Pathogenic study of varicose veins. Angiology 4:59–100

Schmid-Schönbein GW, Takase S, Bergan JJ 2001 New advances in the understanding of the pathophysiology of chronic venous insufficiency. Angiology 52(Suppl 1):S27–S34

Scott HJ, Smith PDC, Scurr JH 1991 Histological study of white blood cells and their association with lipodermatosclerosis and venous ulceration. British Journal of Surgery 78:210–211

Somjen GM 1995 Anatomy of the superficial venous system. Dermatologic Surgery 21:35–45

Takase S, Lerond L, Bergan JJ, Schmid-Schönbein GW 2000 The inflammatory reaction during venous hypertension in the rat. Microcirculation 7:41–52

Takase S, Pascarella L, Lerond L, Bergan JJ, Schmid-Schonbein GW 2004 Venous hypertension, inflammation and valve remodeling. European Journal of Vascular and Endovascular Surgery 28:484–493

Takase S, Schmid-Schönbein G, Bergan JJ 1999 Leukocyte activation in patients with venous insufficiency. Journal of Vascular Surgery 30:148–156

Thomas PR, Nash GB, Dormandy JA 1988 White cell accumulation in dependent legs of patients with venous hypertension: a possible mechanism for trophic changes in the skin. British Medical Journal (Clin Res Ed). 18;296:1693–1695

Weiss RA, Weiss MA 2002 Controlled radiofrequency endovenous occlusion using a unique radiofrequency catheter under duplex guidance to eliminate saphenous varicose vein reflux: A 2-year follow-up. Dermatologic Surgery 28:38–42

Wilkerson LS, Bunker C, Edward JCW, Scurr JH, Coleridge Smith PD 1993 Leukocytes, their role in the etiopathogenesis of skin damage in venous disease. Journal of Vascular Surgery 27:669–675

2 Presentations of Venous Disease

Girish S. Munavalli, Robert A. Weiss

Introduction

Venous disease encompasses a wide spectrum of clinical manifestations, from asymptomatic spider veins on the legs, to intermittently bulging branches of the greater saphenous vein extending across the knee, to dull achy pain in the posterior calf after prolonged standing. The science of treatment of venous disease, phlebology, has roots dating to the ancient Greeks in 400 BC, at which time venous disease was recognized as undesirable and unsightly. Procedures involving the use of instrumentation to traumatize veins were described by Hippocrates in the 4th century BC and procedures such as vein stripping were routinely practiced in the years to follow.

In modern days, venous disease still presents a formidable challenge to diagnose and treat. Venous insufficiency, which is caused by valvular incompetence in the deep or superficial venous system, is the most common form of venous disease. Venous disease affects 40–55% of the population, with common symptoms of leg pain, swelling, and skin changes. Superficial venous insufficiency occurs when a high-pressure leakage develops between the deep and superficial systems, or within the superficial system itself, followed by sequential failure of the venous valves in superficial veins. The two major divisions of the superficial system are the great saphenous vein (GSV) and lesser or small saphenous vein (SSV). Venous insufficiency in this system allows venous blood to escape from its normal flow path and to flow in a retrograde direction down into an already congested leg. Over time, incompetent superficial veins acquire the typical dilated and tortuous appearance of varicosities. Furthermore, insufficiency can lead to chronic morbidity in the form of ulcerative and edematous skin changes in the lower extremities.

Further 'downstream,' changes involving the smaller branching vessels such as unsightly or symptomatic venulectasis and/or telangiectasias, are a major consequence of superficial venous valvular insufficiency. To optimize treatment of varicosities and telangiectasias, pattern recognition of common clinical manifestations is highly recommended. For a regional consideration of the anatomy that gives rise to varices, it is helpful to divide the thigh and calf into eight quadrants: lateral, medial, anterior and posterior (Figs 2.1, 2.2). A regional approach can

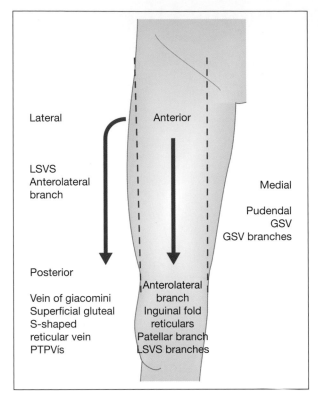

Fig. 2.1 Thigh compartments

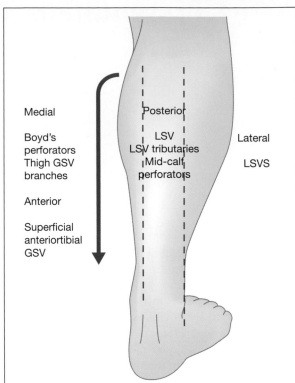

Fig. 2.2 Calf compartments

lead to some unavoidable repetition because many veins extend through many regions or have tributaries that cross many boundaries. Clinical photographs accompanied by simplified diagrams are helpful for identification of the root causes of an unfamiliar pattern of reflux. An understanding of normal venous anatomy is essential for a thorough understanding of venous disease (Figs 2.3, 2.4). Knowledge of the location of the major perforator veins, which connect the deep venous system to the superficial system, is also important for determining the etiology of patterns of varicosities (Fig. 2.5).

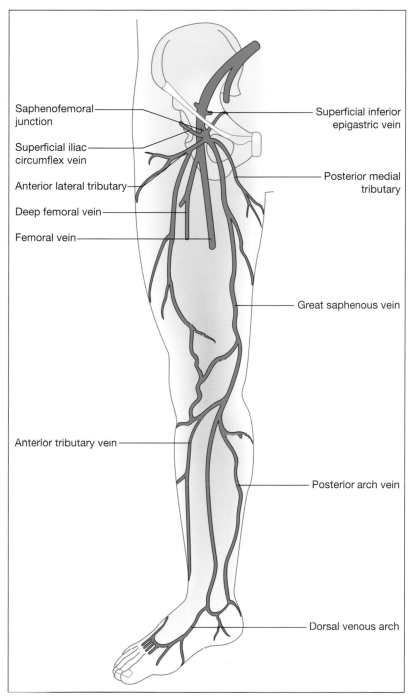

Saphenofemoral junction

Superficial iliac circumflex vein

Anterior lateral tributary

Deep femoral vein

Femoral vein

Anterior tributary vein

Superficial inferior epigastric vein

Posterior medial tributary

Great saphenous vein

Posterior arch vein

Dorsal venous arch

Fig. 2.3 Anterior view of the leg, showing the GSV and its major branches

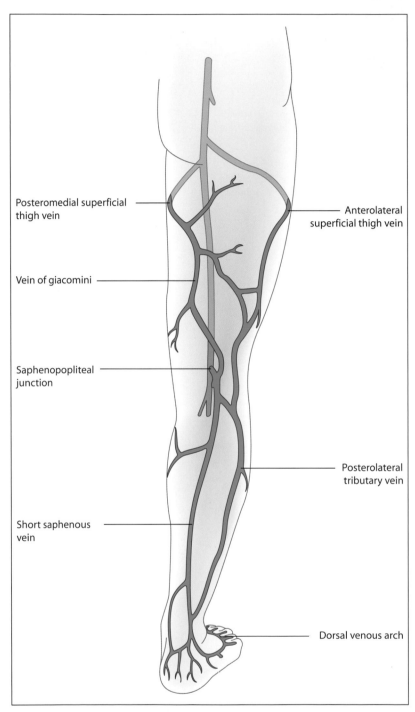

Posteromedial superficial thigh vein

Vein of giacomini

Saphenopopliteal junction

Short saphenous vein

Anterolateral superficial thigh vein

Posterolateral tributary vein

Dorsal venous arch

Fig. 2.4 Posterior view of the leg, showing the LSV and its major branches

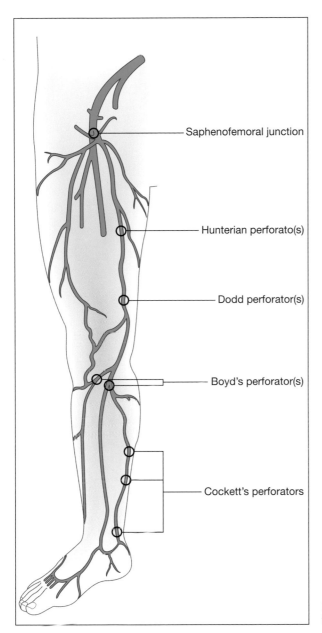

Fig. 2.5 Clinically important perforating veins in the lower extremities

Treatment Approach

It is best to approach the clinical examination of venous disease by visualizing the lower extremities from superior to inferior, starting from the upper thigh to the calf, and concluding with the ankle. Above and below the knee, a division of four compartments can be made in the anterior and posterior planes. When considering the thigh, the presence of reflux in the GSV can manifest in the appearance of varicosities in the medial thigh compartment (Box 2.1).

Thigh quadrants	
Medial thigh	
Incompetent sapheno-femoral junction	Hidden reflux at saphenofemoral junction (only palpable on standing)
Superficial axial branch veins (medial tributaries) of GSV	Resistant telangiectatic matting (just above knee) due to GSV reflux
Distal saccular saphenous vein dilation (just above knee)	
Pudendal vein	Hunterian perforator connection – mid thigh
Posterior thigh	
Superficial gluteal	S-shaped reticular vein of posterior thigh
Posterior thigh perforators emptying into LSVS	S-shaped reticular vein of posterior thigh
Vein of Giacomini	
Lateral thigh	
Lateral subdermic venous system (Albanese) – most common cosmetic pattern	Anterolateral tributary of the GSV
Branch varicosity of lesser saphenous vein	
Anterior thigh	
Antero-lateral tributary of GSV	
Inguinal fold reticulars	Incompetent sapheno-femoral junction
Superficial axial branch veins (lateral tributaries) of GSV	Small anterior branches of the LSVS
Patellar	

Box 2.1 Thigh quadrants

Pudendal veins are 3–4 mm blue reticular varicosities that can be seen extending from the external genitalia. These indicate reflux in the pudendal tributary of the GSV and when they become engorged, as occurs during sexual activity, pain can occur. Treatment of these varicosities is easily accomplished in the absence of saphenofemoral junction incompetence.

Because the GSV typically lies deep and is surrounded by fascial layers, it may be difficult to clinically appreciate prominence that accompanies reflux in this anatomic compartment. In the case of saphenofemoral junction reflux, duplex ultrasound (DUS) is usually necessary to confirm reflux. Prolonged standing may facilitate visualization of the GSV (Fig. 2.6). As the GSV courses distally, superficial tributaries can become varicose as they accept reflux from above and below. In the most distal aspect of the thigh medially, just above the knee, the GSV can emerge from the fascial layers and may become apparent as an enlarged bulbous segment (Fig. 2.7). Clinical mani-

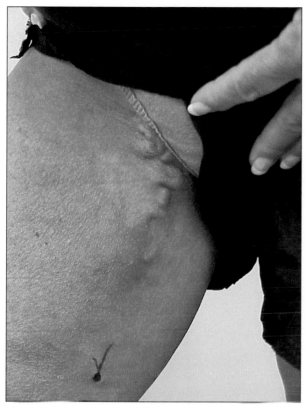

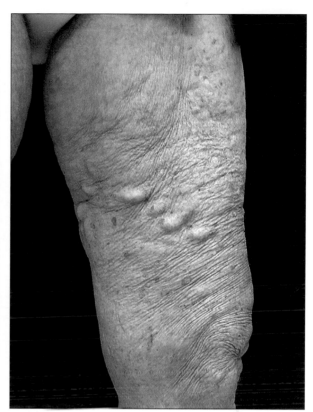

Fig. 2.6 Engorged proximal GSV, resulting from incompetence at the saphenofemoral junction

Fig. 2.7 Saccular dilatations in an enlarged, incompetent GSV

festations of a refluxing GSV can vary based upon the degree of reflux and branch involvement (Fig. 2.8).

Varicose veins in the mid-medial thigh compartment can result from a thigh-perforating vein that communicates between the superficial and deep systems. These can represent incompetence of the so-called Hunterian perforators, or the result of a failed Dodd's perforator from below. Medial thigh telangiectasias situated just above the knee, which prove to be resistant to sclerotherapy, can also be due to a reflux in these perforators and should prompt further evaluation (Fig. 2.9). Persistent telangiectasias along the medial thigh in the distribution of the GSV should prompt an evaluation of the GSV for incompetence (Fig. 2.10).

In the posterior thigh compartment, the most prevalent pattern of superficial venous disease is a central circuitous reticular vein whose origin is in the gluteal region. Often, this vein runs just below the dermis and appears directly below the gluteal fold, and is thought to be a superficial branch of the inferior gluteal vein. Along its length, multiple telangiectasias can arise and prompt patients to seek

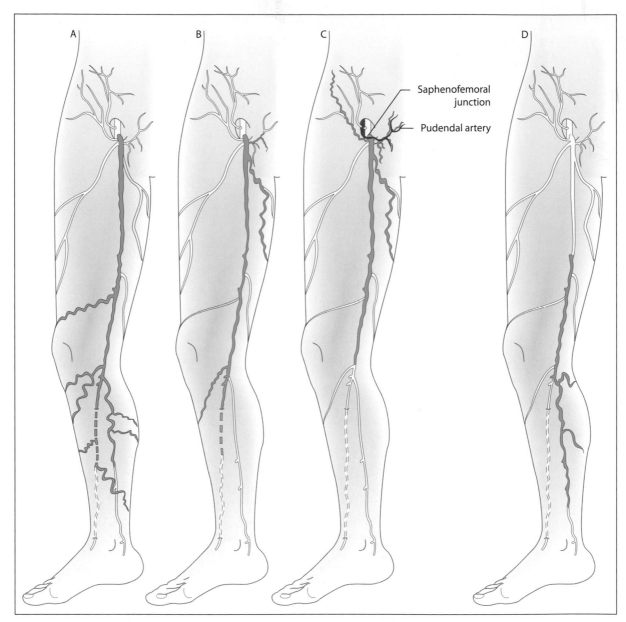

Fig. 2.8 Patterns of GSV reflux in the medial thigh, with and without branch involvement

treatment. Posterior lateral thigh perforating veins (PTPVs) have been shown to dive deep in the posterior thigh and join tributaries of femoral veins (Fig. 2.11). Reticular veins can interconnect with these veins and are quite variable in their position and length. If occurring within 1–2 cm of the popliteal fossa, reflux of the SSV as a contributing factor must be excluded by Doppler/Duplex examination before proceeding with treatment.

An S-shaped reticular vein may be identified as it courses along the posterior thigh. This vein can cause pain with prolonged sitting and

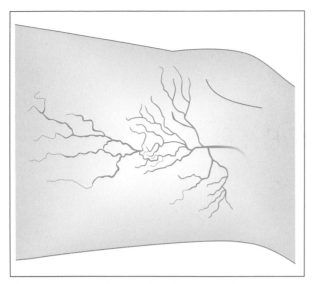

Fig. 2.9 Medial thigh perforator with surrounding telangiectasis

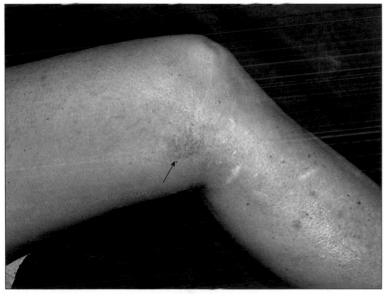

Fig. 2.10 Cluster of persistent telangiectasias resulting from GSV reflux

should be considered as a posterior component of the lateral venous system.

Giacomini vein

The vein of Giacomini is located in the medial part of the posterior thigh compartment and can present with reflux (Fig. 2.12). From a functional point of view, this vein can transmit reflux of the

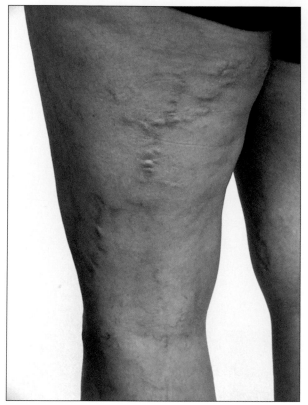

Fig. 2.11 Reflux resulting from PTPVs in a middle-aged female

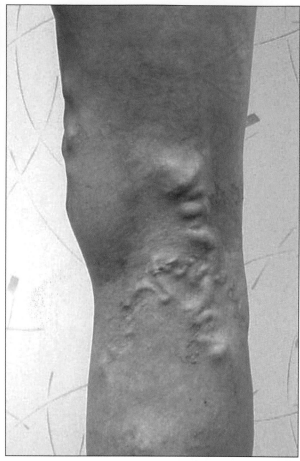

Fig. 2.12 Vein of Giacomini in the posterior thigh compartment

saphenofemoral junction to the lesser saphenous trunk. The lesser saphenous trunk can become secondarily incompetent as a result of this overload. Inversely, reflux of the lesser saphenous network can induce overload of the veins of the greater saphenous network. Very rarely, a badly incompetent GSV itself can be visible on the posterior medial aspect of the thigh, above the knee. More typically a larger vein in this location is a refluxing branch of the GSV.

Lateral subdermic venous system

The classic presentation of venous disease in the lateral thigh is the telangiectatic webs resulting from the lateral subdermic venous system of Albanese (LSVS). Reflux through this stellate network of reticular veins may occur retrograde due to movement of the knee as these veins normally drain by gravity distally rather than the usual pattern of proximal drainage. In young women, the pattern of LSVS reflux most commonly seen is a bridge of telangiectasias associated with a central

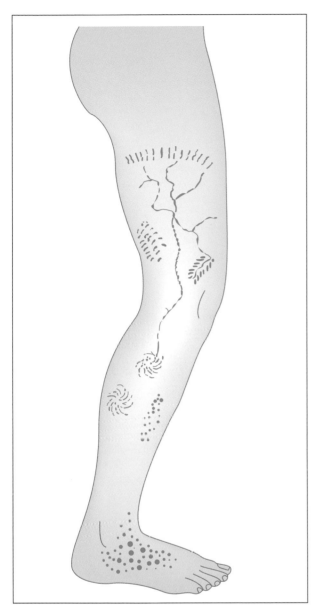

Fig. 2.13 Schematic of the LSVS zone of influence

reticular vein (Fig. 2.13). This clinical pattern must be recognized and treated in its entirety to ensure complete resolution (Fig. 2.14). Consideration should be given to evaluating potential reflux originating at the lateral or posterior knee. Half of the time, however, reflux originates from an incompetent lateral mid-thigh or PTPV. The GSV often gives rise to an anterolateral tributary (ALT) branch that courses laterally along the anterior surface of the thigh. Ultimately, this branch can interact with the LSVS and worsen the clinical manifestation of this system.

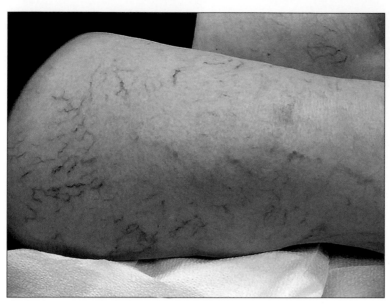

Fig. 2.14 Young female patient presenting with classic LSVS

Veins in the anterior thigh compartment can occasionally arise as a result of GSV reflux. As mentioned earlier, the ALT allows direct communication between the GSV and LSVS. Rarely, a refluxing ALT can occur in an isolated fashion, but usually it is transmitting reflux from the GSV (Fig. 2.15). Near the inguinal area, 3–4 mm varicosities may indicate reflux through a pudendal branch of the GSV. Patellar varicosities often represent a communication between a GSV tributary and reticular veins that communicate with the LSVS.

Veins below the knee

Below the knee, in the calf region, compartments are also similarly arranged (Box 2.2). Varicosities in the posterior compartment usually

Calf quadrants	
Posterior calf	
Lesser saphenous vein	Mid-calf perforator of LSV
LSV major tributaries	LSVS
Greater saphenous vein	
Lateral calf	
Lateral subdermic venous system	
Medial calf	
Boyd's perforators	
Thigh GSV branch reflux	
Anterior calf (pre-tibial)	
Superficial anterior tibial vein	GSV tributaries
GSV	

Box 2.2 Calf quadrants

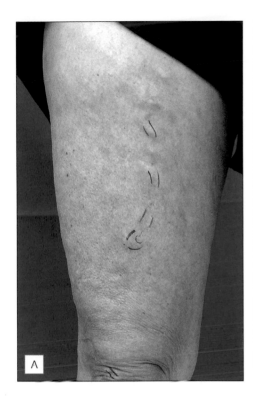

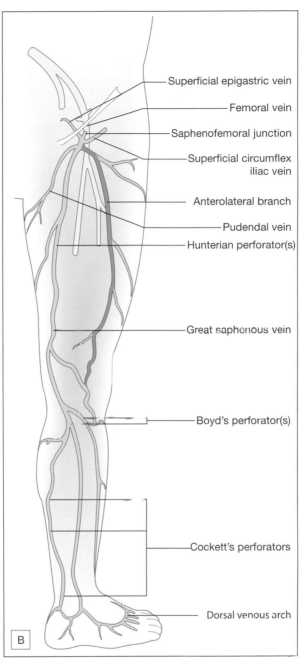

Superficial epigastric vein

Femoral vein

Saphenofemoral junction

Superficial circumflex iliac vein

Anterolateral branch

Pudendal vein

Hunterian perforator(s)

Great saphenous vein

Boyd's perforator(s)

Cockett's perforators

Dorsal venous arch

Fig. 2.15 (**A** and **B**) Isolated reflux in the anterolateral venous branch of the GSV

result from incompetence in the SSV system. Even when refluxing, the SSV is rarely visible along its course from the popliteal fossa, bisecting the two heads of the gastrocnemius muscle on its way to the mid-calf. Doppler or duplex examination is needed to document reflux in this system, if any degree of suspicion is aroused (Fig. 2.16). Care must be taken to rule out contribution from reticular veins of the LSVS in this area. Additionally, major refluxing tributaries of the SSV can manifest lateral to the Achilles tendon. Mid-calf perforators can be distinct from Cockett's perforators and sometimes appear as isolated, bulging in the central calf and are distinctly different from reflux secondary to SSV reflux. Though they have no official name, mid-calf perforators in the posterior compartment are the most common of all calf perforators (Fig. 2.17). LSVS reticular veins can extend onto the posterior calf and must be distinguished from SSV reflux. Lastly, the

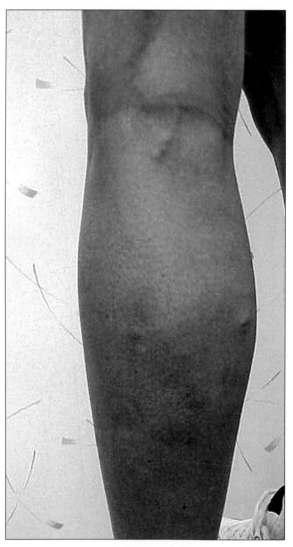

Fig. 2.16 Clinical manifestation of LSV reflux in a young female

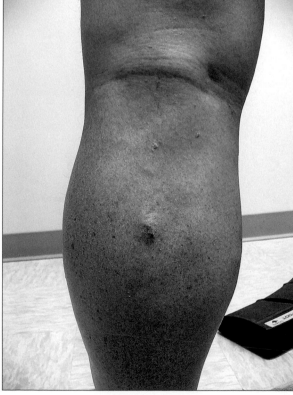

Fig. 2.17 Mid-calf perforator

badly refluxing GSV or a branching tributary can be identified on the posterior medial aspect of the thigh coursing inferiorly onto the calf.

Branches of the LSVS are the dominant presentation of superficial venous disease on the lateral calf. A feeding reticular vein should be identified for effective treatment of this system. If the ALT is communicating with the GSV, this system will appear larger on clinical examination. In the medial calf, GSV incompetence can manifest as a branch varicosity. Visualization of this branch should initiate Doppler/duplex examination of the entire length of the GSV to identify zones of reflux. Perforator-fed varices are also common in this area and have been labeled so-called Boyd's perforators and are thought to exit the superficial fascia and connect the GSV to the crural veins (Fig. 2.18).

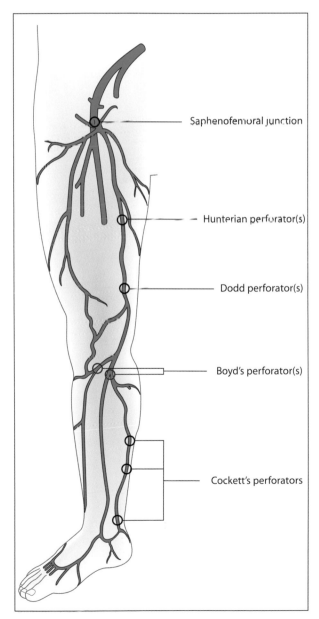

Saphenofemoral junction

Hunterian perforator(s)

Dodd perforator(s)

Boyd's perforator(s)

Cockett's perforators

Fig. 2.18 Common location for Boyd's perforating veins

These veins have been called the most common site for spontaneous occurrence of a primary varicose vein.

In the anterior calf compartment, a superficial anterior tibial reticular vein can demonstrate reflux. Although it drains the GSV medially, it typically occurs in the absence of any reflux in the GSV. This vein can be symptomatic, with spontaneous throbbing occurring when reflux is present. Just superior to the ankle, GSV reflux can be noted as bulging along with a prominence of rope-like tributaries in the area.

The ankle in the anterior calf compartment is seen as a distinct area. Cockett's perforator reflux can present posterior to the medial malleolus as a prelude to deep venous insufficiency. Reflux from both major superficial venous systems can be evident in the ankle area. Advanced SSV reflux is seen primarily in the lateral malleolar area, whereas advanced GSV reflux is seen in the superior-medial malleolar area, and is often associated with skin hyperpigmentation or the development of a bluish stellate telangiectatic/reticular mass known as 'corona phlebectasia' (Fig. 2.19). Finally, the anterior dorsal vein can arise from

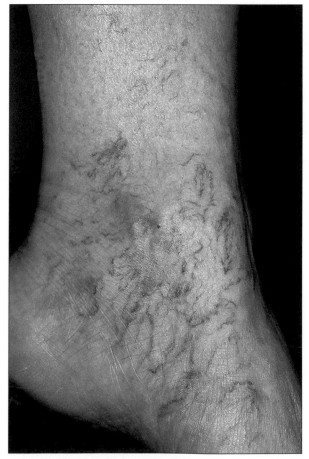

Fig. 2.19 Dense cluster of medial malleolar telangiectasias, known as corona phlebectasia, seen in longstanding GSV reflux

reflux in either system. It traverses across the dorsal ankle to the dorsal venous arch. This vein is a leading candidate for removal via phlebectomy.

Conclusion

With repetition and practice, it is possible to recognize common patterns of abnormal varicose veins and telangiectasias. Recognition is critical for documentation and initial evaluation, however recognition alone is not sufficient to guide treatment. Superficial venous disease of the GSV and SSV can be extremely complex and extremely variable, involving many veins that are not visible on the surface of the skin. Compartmentalization will direct an appropriate examination and diagnostic evaluation, facilitating a correct diagnostic and treatment plan.

Further Reading

Callam MJ 1994 Epidemiology of varicose veins. British Journal of Surgery 81:167–173

Goldman MP 1991 Sclerotherapy: Treatment of varicose and telangiectatic leg veins. Mosby, Baltimore

Weiss RA 1993 Evaluation of the venous system by Doppler ultrasound and photoplethysmography or light reflection rheography before sclerotherapy. Seminars in Dermatology 12:78–87

Weiss RA, Feied CF, Weiss MA 2001 Vein diagnosis and treatment: A comprehensive approach. McGraw-Hill, New York

Weiss RA, Weiss MA 1993 Doppler ultrasound findings in reticular veins of the thigh subdermic lateral venous system and implications for sclerotherapy. Journal of Dermatologic Surgical Oncology 19(10):947–951

Weiss RA, Weiss MA 1995 Continuous wave venous Doppler examination for pretreatment diagnosis of varicose and telangiectatic veins. Dermatologic Surgery 21:58–62

3

Patient Evaluation: History and Physical Examination

Robert A. Weiss

Introduction: Organization of Clinical Examination

The first step is to investigate the patient's presenting complaint and disease history in the context of their general medical and vascular history. The physical examination (including Doppler auscultation) is performed with the patient standing and then in the supine position. The initial assessment culminates with identification of the primary varicose veins and their regions of involvement. Further evaluation is required to quantify functional and esthetic impairment, to assess the risks of possible complications, and to establish a plan for management that will be medically appropriate and acceptable to the patient. The adjunctive utilization of duplex ultrasound (DUS) to formulate this plan is presently considered the standard of care.

History

Evaluation of the patient with varicosities begins with a complete clinical history. This should include general medical and surgical information as well as information about vascular disease. Besides the presenting complaint, it is important to document the time of onset of the symptoms and signs of venous difficulty and the clinical progression of the disease, including the rapidity of such progression. Exacerbating factors should also be recorded. The patient should be questioned about each of the symptoms known to be associated with venous insufficiency; leg heaviness, exercise intolerance, pain or tenderness along the course of a vein, pruritus, 'restless' legs, night cramps, edema, and paresthesias.

Presenting Complaint

Patients may consult a dermatologic surgeon because of troublesome symptoms or esthetic concerns. They may desire advice on the medical implications of varicose veins or be interested in therapy, especially nonsurgical methods of treatment. Some visits are prompted by the recent onset of complications, such as the rupture of a varicose vein with subsequent bleeding or the development of dermatitis, thrombophlebitis, cellulitis, or ulceration. Treatment that does not properly address the patient's primary concerns will not result in a satisfactory overall outcome. Patients also need to have a thorough understanding that long hours of standing without support can stimulate the formation of new veins.

General History

The following categories of information regarding general medical history should be obtained for each patient:

- Sex, age, weight, and height
- Medical history, including hypertension, diabetes, allergy history, tobacco consumption, rheumatological history, and general disease
- Surgical history, including any fractures or surgical operations
- Gynecological and obstetric history, including the number of pregnancies and miscarriages, plan for future pregnancies, duration, dosage, and effect on venous complaints of hormone replacement therapy or oral contraception, and any variation of symptoms with the menstrual cycle.

History of Vascular Disease

A more detailed history of pre-existing vascular disease, including venous and arterial disease, and prior vascular events, should also be recorded, including:

- History of venous insufficiency, including the date of onset of visible abnormal vessels and the date of onset of any symptoms
- Presence or absence of predisposing factors such as heredity, trauma to the legs, occupational prolonged standing or sports participation
- History of edema, including the date of onset, predisposing factors, site, intensity, hardness, and modification after a night's rest
- History of any prior evaluation of or treatment for venous disease, including medications, injections, surgery, or compression
- History of superficial or deep thrombophlebitis, including the date of onset, site, predisposing factors, and sequelae
- History of any other vascular disease, including peripheral arterial disease, coronary artery disease, lymphedema, or lymphangitis
- Family history of vascular disease of any type.

Active Symptoms

Symptoms of venous disease are most often localized to the medial aspect of the leg. Symptoms are often intensified by heat, prolonged standing, or concurrent menstruation in women in whom progesterone secretion is predominant. Venous symptoms are typically relieved by cold, ambulation, rest with leg elevation, or wearing of graded pressure elastic stockings.

Characteristics of venous pain include a dull ache, burning or pruritis. This pain may be localized to a protruding varicose or reticular vein. It is rarely described as a sharp stabbing pain or pain radiating down the back of the thigh. Surprisingly, nighttime muscle cramping may be instigated by venous insufficiency as many patients relate that the cramping is eliminated when varicose veins are treated by endovenous techniques. Restless legs may rarely be caused by venous insufficiency. The extent and origin of venous disease and pain are listed in Box 3.1.

Physical Examination/Clinical Assessment

Findings of special importance on physical examination are listed in Box 3.2. Some of these physical findings may help to guide the choice of treatment modality and predict the expected degree of difficulty in implementing this successfully. Ambulatory phlebectomy of thick-walled veins is time consuming and tedious but effective as this type of vein may be resistant to sclerotherapy. Endovenous techniques using new small fiberoptic delivery systems are being actively investigated as a treatment option for this situation.

Clinical evaluation of the patient with venous disease remains the foundation for subsequent diagnostic and therapeutic interventions. The presenting complaint and the patient's goals for treatment must be defined and clearly understood. Knowledge of the patient's medical, social, work and family environment is also important. A general assessment of the patient's venous disease, including its severity and consequences, is critical for estimating the risk of disease-associated complications, both vascular (superficial venous thrombosis, prehemorrhagic bulla, ulceration) and trophic (eczema, cellulitis, leg ulcers).

For example, swelling may result from acute venous obstruction (such as is seen in deep vein thrombosis [DVT]), or from deep or superficial venous reflux, or other nonvenous causes. Hepatic insufficiency, renal failure, cardiac decompensation, infection, trauma, and environmental effects can all produce lower extremity pitting edema that may be indistinguishable from the edema of venous obstruction or venous insufficiency. Edema due to lymphatic system malfunction may be due to primary obstruction of lymphatic outflow.

Rather than being considered a special diagnostic modality, the use of Doppler for auscultation is considered an integral part of the clinical examination of patients with venous disease. It is equivalent to the stethoscope in a routine physical examination. Hand-held Doppler helps to confirm the clinical findings of the physical examination, and is particularly valuable because it can reveal relevant subsurface reflux in portions of the greater saphenous vein that cannot be visualized. Doppler helps define the topography of varicose disease and the hemodynamic status of the deep venous system. Repeated examinations over time help to document the results of treatment or the natural course of the disease.

Equipment

The clinical examination requires a medical file, an examination platform, excellent lighting, a phlebological examination table, continuous-

Venous symptoms

- 50% of females
- 20% of males
- Many women deprive themselves of outdoor activity
- More than cosmetic for many
- Leads to aching, fatigue, redness, itching, swelling, and ulceration
- Overwhelmingly underdiagnosed cause of leg pain in women

Box 3.1 Venous symptoms

Physical examination findings associated with venous reflux

- Asymmetry of limbs
- Size, length, and ankle diameter
- Scars
- Previous venous surgery
- Previous venous ulcers
- Cutaneous signs of chronic venous insufficiency
- Superficial vascular malformations such as port wine stains
- Muscular tone and development
- Hypertrophy of veins and thickening of vein walls

Box 3.2 Physical examination findings associated with venous reflux

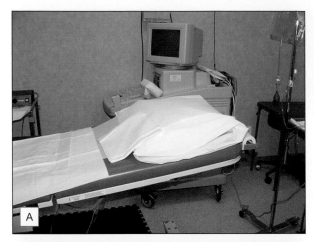

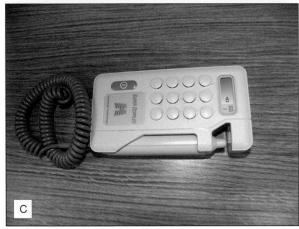

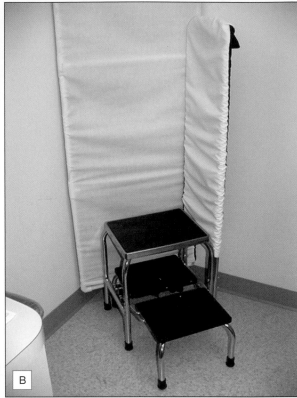

Fig. 3.1 (**A**) An examination table tilted in reverse Trendelenburg to allow for examination of reflux. (**B**) The examination platform. (**C**) The hand-held Doppler device

wave Doppler apparatus, and a small amount of miscellaneous equipment (Fig. 3.1).

Examination platform

Having the patient stand on a platform consisting of two or three steps will greatly increase the physical comfort for the physician and allow a more complete examination. While on a platform, the patient can be examined in a standing position without requiring the physician to contort or excessively extend the neck.

Lighting

Lighting should be even and consistent. The simplest approach is to have a 75 W lamp on each side of the patient. Uniform overhead fluorescent lighting is satisfactory. Hot spots from strong halogen lamps will bleach out smaller blue reticular veins and such lamps are therefore not recommended. Useful devices to examine smaller telangiectasias without surface reflection of light include several cross-polarized visualization systems manufactured by Syris Scientific

(LLC, Grey, MA). The visual enhancement of fine telangiectasias and hard-to-see reticular veins permitted by these devices is seen in Figure 3.2. Transillumination using LED or halogen light sources (see www.veinlite.com) may be helpful to map out reticular veins within 1–2 mm of the skin surface (Fig. 3.3).

Examination table

The examination table can be simple and inexpensive, but should allow examination of the patient either in a half-seated or totally supine position. A hydraulic examination table will facilitate the examination by permitting the patient to be raised to a level convenient for the examiner and to be tilted into Trendelenburg and reverse Trendelenburg positions as needed. A hydraulic table will also be useful for subsequent treatments and help to protect the neck and spine of the treating physician (Fig. 3.4).

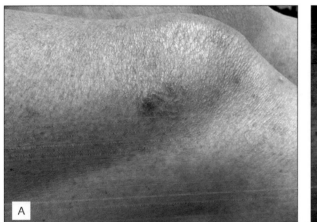 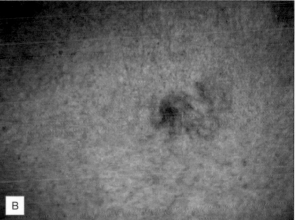

Fig. 3.2 Enhancement of view of telangiectasia. (**A**) View with normal fluorescent lighting. (**B**) View with Syris v600

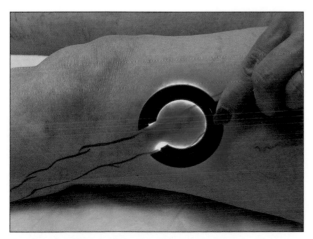

Fig. 3.3 Transillumination of a reticular varicosity

Maximum Vessel Dilation

30° reverse trendelenburg

the VasScan™ Table

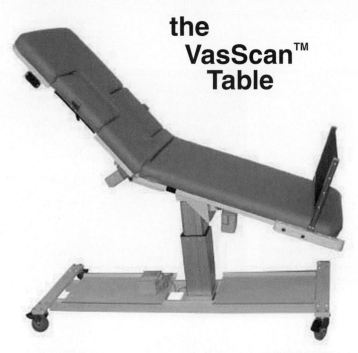

the ONLY vascular specific exam table

Upper Extremity Armboard
(optional)

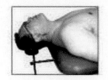

Carotid Head Support
(optional)

Additional Options
- Positioning SafeTwedges
- Rigid or collapsible safety rails
- Paper roll holder & cutter
- Storage trays
- 74 Optional vinyl colors

Fig. 3.4 Examination table brochure for a Trendelenburg table

Doppler apparatus

The 'continuous-wave Doppler' examination is the simplest, least expensive, and most rapid method by which to enhance the physical examination of patients with chronic venous insufficiency. Provided it is performed by an experienced operator with a good knowledge of pathophysiology and venous anatomical variants, this is a useful adjunct to the visual and tactile examination.

Physical Examination (Standing)

This examination is initially performed with the patient standing, and then portions are repeated with the patient in the supine or prone position. The upright position corresponds to the position of maximal venous dilatation, while in the supine position the effect of hydrostatic pressure disappears and varicose veins collapse. As mentioned, the physical examination begins with inspection, palpation and percussion, followed by Doppler auscultation. It is not uncommon for patients to feel lightheaded or even to faint while undergoing this examination. A cool room, particularly for patients with a previous history of vasovagal reactions, will help to minimize this risk. Patients should be warned to alert the physician immediately if they are feeling faint.

Inspection

Inspection is performed in an organized way from distal to proximal and from anterior to posterior, with the patient positioned on the highest step of the exam platform. Lighting should be even, without any zones of shadow. The examination is bilateral, with comparison of findings on each leg. In addition to the legs, the perineal region, pubic region and abdominal wall must also be examined. The presence of a female chaperone for examination of female patients is highly recommended.

Inspection should be sufficient to detect morphological abnormalities such as an abnormally large toe, swollen leg, hourglass leg, knee joint alignment abnormalities, or lengthening or trophic changes of one lower limb compared to the other. Further inspection should identify any cutaneous disorders, such as (1) ulceration; (2) telangiectasias of the leg, foot or ankle; (3) acrocyanosis; (4) eczema; (5) brown spots; (6) ochre dermatitis; (7) flat angiomata; (8) prominent varicose veins (small, large, rectilinear, or tortuous); (9) scars from a prior surgical operation; (10) or evidence of previous sclerosant injections. Particular attention must be made to identify any venous dilatations within the perineal, suprapubic, or abdominal regions.

Normal veins are typically visibly distended at the foot and ankle, and occasionally in the popliteal fossa. For other regions of the leg, visible distention usually implies disease. Translucent skin may allow normal veins to be visible as a light blue subdermal reticular pattern, but numerous dilated veins at or above the ankle usually are evidence of venous pathology (Fig. 3.5).

One of the primary goals of inspection is to determine the predominant 'zone of influence' of involvement. The examiner must

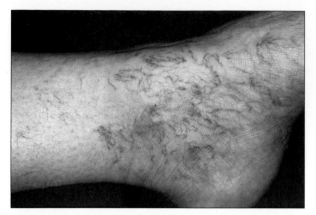

Fig. 3.5 Telangiectatic groups at the ankle indicative of venous disease in the great saphenous vein

consider whether the veins arise from regions of the great saphenous vein (GSV), short saphenous vein (SSV) or lateral venous system. Darkened, discolored, stained skin is often a sign of chronic venous stasis, particularly if localized along the medial ankle and the medial aspect of the lower leg. As these areas require drainage from a competent GSV that is, along with its attached perforating veins, fully patent along its entire length, they are particularly susceptible to GSV malfunction. Nonhealing ulcers in this area are also most likely due to underlying venous stasis. Skin changes or ulcers that are localized only to the lateral aspect of the ankle are much more likely to be related to prior trauma or arterial insufficiency than to pure venous insufficiency.

The appearance of new varices and telangiectasias often is noted during pregnancy. Venous outflow obstruction from uterine compression of the pelvic outflow tracts was once thought to be responsible, but it has been shown that this is an uncommon mechanism for the development of varicose veins of pregnancy. It is now believed that most of the effect is due to both hormonal changes, which render the vein wall and the valves themselves more pliable, and the increased circulating blood volume. Veins of the leg act as a reservoir for the increased blood volume and expand accordingly. The sudden appearance of new dilated varicosities during pregnancy still warrants a full evaluation for the possibility of acute DVT, which may occur during pregnancy.

Light palpation

Light palpation is often performed as a part of the process of inspection. The entire surface of the skin is gently pressed with the fingertips, because dilated veins may be palpable even where they are not readily seen. Palpation helps to locate both normal and abnormal veins, but it sometimes is possible to distinguish the soft collapsibility of a normal vein from the 'distended inner tube' sensation of a varicosity. Palpation is only useful while the patient is standing.

After a few minutes of standing, in some thin patients the arch of the long saphenous vein may be felt, especially when reflux is present at the junction. This finding is best appreciated two fingerbreadths below the inguinal ligament and just medial to the femoral artery. In patients with saphenofemoral incompetence, a forced coughing maneuver may produce a palpable thrill or sudden expansion at this level. The short saphenous vein is often more difficult to examine manually, but it may be felt in the popliteal fossa in some slender patients after a period of standing or when involved with reflux. Other normal superficial veins above the feet should not be palpable even after prolonged standing.

Deep palpation

Palpation of an area of leg pain or tenderness may reveal a firm, thickened thrombosed vein. These palpable thrombosed vessels are virtually always superficial veins. However it cannot be assumed that an apparent isolated superficial thrombosis is benign, since such superficial venous thrombosis commonly occurs in combination with less easily detected deep thrombosis. A completely thrombosed popliteal vein may sometimes be palpated in the popliteal fossa, and the same is true of the common femoral vein at the groin. Palpation for deep thrombosis is not reliable since the vast majority of cases of DVT do not produce any abnormality that can be appreciated, even with firm tactile pressure.

The presence of significant obesity or edema may make the underlying varicose veins difficult to palpate. Sometimes varices may be more readily palpable after edema has been reduced by a few minutes of compression with a blood pressure cuff. A muscular hernia can simulate a varicose vein on palpation, but the two can be distinguished because muscular herniae usually are situated in the anterolateral compartment of the leg. Hernias, not veins, will collapse on standing and during forced flexion of the foot on the leg.

Percussion

Percussion, an older diagnostic technique, can be used to trace out the course of veins already detected on palpation, discover varicose veins that could not be palpated, and assess the relationships between the various varicose vein networks.

The patient stands, and a vein segment suspected of containing incompetent valves is tapped at one point while an examining hand feels for a 'pulse wave' at another point. The propagation of a palpable pulse wave demonstrates a patent superficial venous segment with incompetent valves connecting the two positions. The examination must be carried out with caution, because prolonged standing will cause even a normal vein to become distended, and if valves have floated open, a pulse wave may be propagated even in the absence of pathology. The technique is most valuable when a large bulging venous cluster in the lower leg has no obvious connection with a varicosity in the upper thigh, yet palpable pulse wave propagation between the two demonstrates the existence of an unseen connection.

Veins and their connections become gradually better defined through inspection, palpation, and percussion to form a 'venous map' that will later guide treatment. The courses of all the dilated veins that are identified may be marked along the leg with a pen, and later transcribed into the medical record as a map of all known areas of superficial reflux. A photograph of this penned map may be taken as well. This preliminary evaluation will be confirmed, more precisely defined, and completed through Doppler auscultation.

Doppler auscultation

The physical examination as described thus far can locate areas of venous dilatation, but it cannot distinguish between dilated veins of normal function or true varicosities that carry venous blood in a retrograde direction. Doppler examination is the easiest method by which to distinguish incompetent refluxing varicose veins from large veins that carry antegrade flow.

Doppler ultrasound is named after Austrian physicist Johann Christian Doppler, who in 1842 explained the significance of an apparent increase or decrease in the frequency of waves emitted or reflected from an object that is moving toward or away from the observer. The essence of the principle is this: when the object is moving toward the observer, each wave is emitted or reflected from a position a little closer than the one before, thus each wave comes back a little sooner than expected, and the frequency appears to be higher. When the object is moving away from the observer, each wave comes back a little later than it would if the object were not moving, so the frequency appears to be lower.

When used as part of the physical examination, Doppler auscultation is performed with the upper hand holding the Doppler transducer along the axis of a vein to be examined, with the probe at an angle of 45 degrees to the skin. If there are obviously dilated veins that have the appearance of varicosities, gentle tapping on the underlying vessels produces a strong Doppler signal and confirms the correct positioning of the transducer. The lower (or distal) hand then performs 'augmentation' by compressing and then releasing the underlying veins and muscles below the level of the probe. Compression causes forward flow in the direction of the valves, and release causes backward flow through incompetent valves, but no signal is detected if the valves are competent and the blood cannot flow backwards. These distal compression–decompression maneuvers are repeated while gradually ascending the limb to a level where the reflux can no longer be appreciated.

When telangiectasias are noted on the lateral surface of the thigh, the Doppler may be able to demonstrate reflux in feeding reticular veins that originate around the knee. If there are no visible or palpable dilated varices, the presence or absence of retrograde flow is assessed at the top, middle and bottom of the long and short saphenous veins on each leg.

Doppler probes of different frequencies are used depending on the depth of the vessels to be examined, because lower frequency ultrasound penetrates deeper through tissues before being reflected back to the transducer. A Doppler probe that emits frequencies of 8–10 MHz is best suited to examining vessels that are < 2.0 cm deep, although it has been found difficult to hear reflux > 1 cm below the skin surface with these frequencies. Deeper vessels up to 4 cm deep may be examined using a 5 MHz probe.

From the saphenofemoral junction, the Doppler transducer is gradually moved several centimeters below the inguinal ligament following the course of the GSV. If the vein can be seen or palpated in this region, the probe can be placed by feel. Otherwise, the probe should be moved along the vein by following the sound of flow (whether spontaneous flow or flow augmented with compression). Distal compression and release should produce a transient increase in signal followed by rapid cessation of flow as competent valves snap shut. Flow during proximal compression or after release of distal compression is a sign of valvular incompetence and reflux.

In the normal patient, a Valsalva maneuver (increasing intra-abdominal pressure by taking a deep breath and 'bearing down' with the abdominal muscles as if trying to defecate) causes forward flow to cease within a half-second as the valve shuts at the saphenofemoral junction. Because the veins are large at this level, reflux appears as a 'hurricane' or 'windstorm' sound, indicating reverse flow that appears during Valsalva or as 'rebound reflux' immediately after cessation of distal compression. If the transducer is positioned directly over the saphenofemoral junction, reflux indicates incompetent valves at the junction (Fig. 3.6).

The Doppler examination adds a vast quantity of information to the physical examination, but it is not an actual imaging study. When there is any uncertainty about the physical examination or Doppler findings, DUS must be performed. With small DUS devices, some now argue that use of duplex should be the initial step and Doppler examination may be superfluous or redundant.

Physical Examination (Supine Position)

After the standing examination, the patient is placed in the supine position on the examining table in order to carry out an examination without venous filling. When a patient is in the supine or prone position, the superficial vessels are empty, thus neither percussion nor Doppler auscultation provide any useful diagnostic information. However, the deep venous system remains full when the patient is supine, and Doppler examination of the deep veins is best carried out with the patient in this position.

Inspection and light palpation

Each limb is again inspected, starting with the toes and moving proximally to the plantar arch, dorsum and surfaces of the feet, ankle, leg, knee, thigh, groin, and lesser pelvis. This inspection should detect

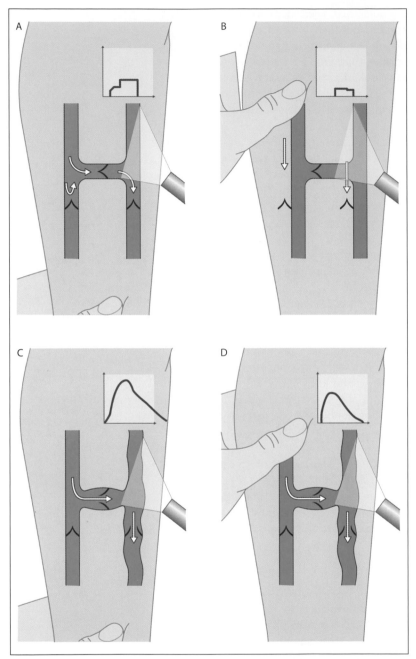

Fig. 3.6 Proximal and distal compression Doppler ultrasound examination. *Of competent perforator valves*: (**A**) During proximal compression, a brief sound is heard, which rapidly concludes as blood movement is stopped by competent valves. (**B**) During distal compression, brief normal forward flow is heard. As distal compression is released, blood flows backwards under gravity but is rapidly stopped by competent valves. *Of incompetent perforator valves*: (**C**) During proximal compression, a long sound is heard as blood movement is detected through a wide-open incompetent valve. The sound continues as long as compression is applied. As compression is released, flow stops. (**D**) During distal compression, a brief normal upward flow is heard, however as distal compression is released, blood flow continues backwards with a prolonged sound, as incompetent valves are unable to prevent continued flow propelled by hydrostatic pressure (gravity). Deflections of the sound graph may be oriented in either direction; here flow towards the transducer is shown as negative while flow away from the transducer is shown as positive

interdigital mycosis, plantar callus, micro-ulcers on the edges of an area of 'atrophie blanche,' and other small problems that may have been missed in the standing examination. If signs of pigmentation in association with stasis dermatitis, ulceration, or any other trophic disorder are observed, the lesions should be measured and photographed. At this time distal and proximal arterial pulses are palpated. An ankle-brachial index is obtained if there is any suspicion of arterial insufficiency.

Deep palpation

Deep palpation with the patient in the supine position is useful to assess the texture of the deep subcutaneous planes and to detect the presence of edema, cellulitis, arteriovenous fistulas, and abnormal lymph nodes.

Edema above the level of the toes is detected by applying gentle and prolonged pressure with the thumb, which sinks as far as the underlying hard plane (the medial surface of the tibia, for example). The amount and extent of edema are documented by measuring the leg with a tape measure at the narrowest part of the ankle, at the widest part of the leg, and at a point 10 cm above the superior margin of the patella.

Complementary Clinical Maneuvers

Several traditional maneuvers are useful to help demonstrate classic venous pathophysiology, but none are reliable enough to displace the Doppler examination, which is far more reliable.

Trendelenburg's test

A classic physical examination maneuver, this test may distinguish patients whose distal venous congestion is caused by superficial venous reflux from patients whose problem is caused by incompetence of the valves within the deep venous system. To perform the Trendelenburg test, the leg is elevated until the congested superficial veins have all collapsed. A tourniquet (or the examiner's hand) is used to occlude a vein at a point of suspected reflux from the deep system into the superficial varicosity. Most often the greater saphenous vein is manually occluded just below the saphenofemoral junction at the groin, but any large vein may be investigated in a similar manner. The patient is made to stand, with the occlusion still in place. If the distal varicosity remains more or less empty, or fills very slowly, then the occluding hand or tourniquet is suddenly removed. Sudden dilation of the varicosity means that the principal entry point of high pressure into the superficial system has been correctly identified. Rapid filling of the varicosity despite manual occlusion of the suspected high point of reflux means that another reflux pathway is involved. If the filling is unusually rapid, it usually means that deep vein valves are incompetent between the groin and the level at which the reflux 'escapes' the deep system (through an incompetent perforating vein) into the superficial system.

Further Clinical Assessment

Examination of the arterial system, particularly of the lower limbs, consists of manual detection of peripheral pulses as well as palpation and auscultation of the arteries. Additionally, Doppler is used to measure the systolic blood pressure at the ankle and elbow to determine an ankle-brachial index. Clinical assessment may also include evaluation of the osteoarticular system, particularly the joints at the ankles, knees, and hips, as well as a sensory and deep tendon reflex evaluation of the neurological system.

Charting

Preliminary assessment

A preliminary assessment is an important guide to determine subsequent management, and must clarify a number of interrelated issues and ascertain specific pathologies:

- The severity of the functional and esthetic impairment
- The diagnosis of essential varicose veins
- The patency and valvular competency of the deep venous system
- The absence of deep system angiodysplasia
- The topography of all varicose lesions
- The topography of the great and short saphenous veins
- The degree of tissue sequelae
- The possible need for additional investigations to confirm, refute, or complete the diagnosis, or to guide the choice of treatment.

Classification and quantification

A consensus document defines two alternative classification schemes for patients with venous disease: patients may be classified either by the type of chronic venous insufficiency or by the severity of the varicose disease. This classification system of venous disorders is based upon clinical, etiological, anatomical and pathophysiological data (CEAP classification). Each category is assigned a number according to a scale. The total value assigns a clinical stage of chronic venous disease (CVD).

An alternative system is a varicose disease scoring system that is based on the maximum clinical diameter (MCD) as determined by palpation and measurement by calipers or tape measure after digital detection of the vessel margins. A Clinical Identification Grid is constructed by taking into account for each limb the MCD of each of the great saphenous, short saphenous, and nonsaphenous territories. This grid can be used to follow the course of the varicose disease in a quantitative fashion and to conduct studies on patients with a comparable varicose state.

Summary

The initial evaluation will include an appropriate clinical consultation, including a description of the main presenting complaint and its history, the history of venous and other diseases, and any prior treatments together with their results. The results of complete inspection, detailed palpation, careful percussion and Doppler auscultation are then recorded. It is helpful to use a standard drawing of the lower limbs to map the precise location of varicose dilatations and the information provided by auscultation. Other physical findings, such as the margins of a leg ulcer, can also be indicated on the same drawing. This type of assessment allows a precise mapping of positive venous findings, thus facilitating evaluation of the current and long-term risks of venous insufficiency. It is important to document all relevant information, such as the presenting complaint, history, symptoms and signs, and to preserve in a file a detailed set of anatomical and venodynamic diagrams. Collective assessment and interpretation of all this data allows the formulation of an appropriate management program for each patient.

Further reading

Kistner RL, Eklof B, Masuda EM 1996 Diagnosis of chronic venous disease of the lower extremities: the 'CEAP' classification [see comments]. Mayo Clinic Proceedings 71:338–345

McMullin GM, Smith PDC, Scurr JH 1991 A study of tourniquets in the investigation of venous insufficiency. Phlebology 6:133–139

Perthes G 1895 Uber die Operation der Unterschenkelvaricen nach Trendelenburg. Deutsch Med Wehrschr 21: 252. 1895.

Santler R 1969 Venous insufficiency and its recognition in practice. Z Haut Geschlechtskr 44:699–706

Schultz Ehrenburg U, Hubner H-J 1989 Reflux diagnosis with Doppler ultrasound (monograph). Schattauer, Stuttgart, New York

Sherman RS 1964 Varicose veins: anatomy re-evaluation of Trendelenburg tests and operating procedure. Surgical Clinics of North America 44:1369–1369

Sparey C, Haddad N, Sissons G, Rosser S, De Cossart L 1999 The effect of pregnancy on the lower-limb venous system of women with varicose veins. European Journal of Vascular and Endovascular Surgery 18:294–299

Weiss RA 1993 Evaluation of the venous system by Doppler ultrasound and photoplethysmography or light reflection rheography before sclerotherapy. Seminars in Dermatology 12:78–87

Weiss RA, Duffy D 1999 Clinical benefits of lightweight compression: Reduction of venous-related symptoms by ready-to-wear lightweight gradient compression hosiery. Dermatologic Surgery 25:701–704

Weiss RA, Feied CF, Weiss MA 2001 Vein Diagnosis and Treatment: A comprehensive approach. McGraw-Hill

Weiss RA, Weiss MA 1993 Doppler ultrasound findings in reticular veins of the thigh subdermic lateral venous system and implications for sclerotherapy. Journal of Dermatological Surgery and Oncology 19:947–951

Weiss RA, Weiss MA 1995 Continuous wave venous Doppler examination for pretreatment diagnosis of varicose and telangiectatic veins. Dermatologic Surgery 21:58–62

4

An Overview of Therapy for Leg Veins

Jeffrey T.S. Hsu

Introduction

Depending on the size and location of the leg veins to be treated, any of a multitude of therapeutic options may be appropriate. While selecting the correct treatment techniques is important, management of patient expectations prior to the treatment can be equally vital. A standard list of topics should be discussed with every prospective patient (Box 4.1). The patient must understand that although improvement is expected, there is no guarantee regarding this or the degree of improvement. Risks accompany any medical procedure, and these must be discussed thoroughly. Once the physician has conveyed the necessary information, the patient should be encouraged to ask questions and should be provided with a detailed explanation of any concerns, as appropriate. If the patient appears overly anxious, overly demanding, or simply unable to understand the procedure, the patient may not be an ideal candidate for intervention.

Topics of pre-treatment discussion with patient

- Patient expectations
- Expected discomfort during treatment
- Benefits of treatment
- Possible complications of treatment
- Treatment alternatives
- Post-treatment care
- Duration and nature of recovery phase

Box 4.1 Topics of pre-treatment discussion with patient

Compression

Use of external compression therapy (CT) is a fundamental strategy in the treatment of lower extremity venous disease. Despite recent therapeutic advancements in leg vein treatment, compression remains a simple, effective, and inexpensive modality. It should be considered as the primary treatment in many conditions, and as an adjunct when other treatments are employed (Box 4.2).

Active and Passive Compression

Compression can be either passive or active. Passive compression is applied using inelastic bandages. As muscles contract, the bandages resist the volume increase and thereby increased pressure is delivered. As the muscles relax, the volume decreases so that minimal pressure is applied by the bandages. On the other hand, active compression using elastic bandages permits application of pressure both during muscular exercise and at rest. This constant pressure may not be tolerated by bedridden or inactive patients, and may be contraindicated in arterial insufficiency (Fig. 4.1).

Indications for leg vein compression

- DVT prophylaxis
- Symptomatic varicose veins
- Chronic venous insufficiency
- Venous ulcers
- Post sclerotherapy
- Post phlebectomy
- Pregnancy
- Thrombophlebitis
- Active DVT treatment

Box 4.2 Indications for leg vein compression

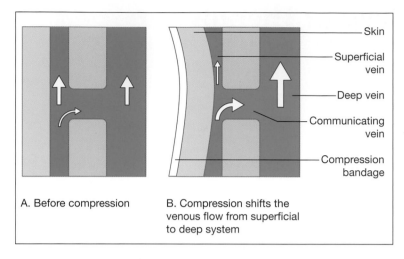

A. Before compression

B. Compression shifts the
venous flow from superficial
to deep system

Fig. 4.1 (**A**) Before compression.
(**B**) Compression shifts the venous
flow from superficial to deep
system

Whether passive or active, compression improves venous disease through several mechanisms. Compression narrows the lumens of the veins in the superficial system, which accelerates venous flow, decreases venous pooling, and helps to shift venous flow from the superficial into the deep venous system. Compression also may partially restore valvular function, and gradually reverse degenerative changes in the veins, thus also reducing venous reflux.

Compression Bandages (Tables 4.1 and 4.2; Fig. 4.2)

Short-stretch bandages

Various modalities are available for compression. Completely rigid inelastic bandages, like the zinc gel Unna boot (Unna-Flex, Convatec, Princeton, NJ), and the Gelocast (Beiersdorf Inc., Norwalk, CT), both dry to form a cast around the leg. Short-stretch bandages such as Comprilan (Beiersdorf, Norwalk, CT) are made of fabric that stretches

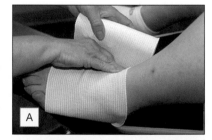
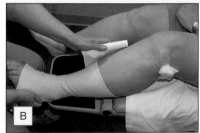
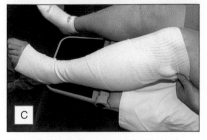

Fig. 4.2 (**A–C**) Proper application of stretch bandage post sclerotherapy

Manufacturers of compression stockings	
Brand	**Location and Telephone number**
Jobst	Charlotte, NC 1-704-554-9933
Sigvaris	Branford, CT 1-800-322-7744
JuZo	Cuyahoga Falls, OH 1-800-222-4999
Medi	Arlington Heights, IL 1-800-633-6334
Venosan	Asheboro, NC 1-910-672-6062

Table 4.1 Manufacturers of compression stockings

Manufacturers of compression bandages		
Manufacturer	**Type**	**Adherence/Name**
Se Pro Healthcare Montgomery, PA	High Stretch	Nonhesive/Tubigrip
Beiersdorf Norwalk, CT	Low Stretch	Nonhesive/Comprilan Cohesive/Comprihaft Adhesive/Elastoplast
Beiersdorf	High Stretch	Nonhesive/Eloflex Cohesive/Elohaft
Beiersdorf	Non-Stretch	Cohesive/Gelocast
3M Health Care St. Paul, MN	High Stretch	Adhesive/Microfoam
Convatec Princeton, NJ	Non-Stretch	Cohesive/Unna-Flex
Conco Medical Bridgeport, CT	Low Stretch	Cohesive/Medi-Rip

Table 4.2 Manufacturers of compression bandages

30–50%. Inelastic bandages and short-stretch bandages exert passive compression to treat edema, deep vein thrombosis (DVT), or ulcerations due to chronic venous insufficiency (CVI). They must be applied by trained staff to ensure a proper fit and remain in place for several days continuously. However, as edema remits and leg circumference decreases, the inelastic nature of the bandages fails to accommodate for this change and corresponding pressure loss can occur as early as within the first few hours of application.

Long-stretch bandages

Long-stretch bandages, made of fabric that can stretch 100–200%, provide active compression, indicated after surgery, sclerotherapy, or thrombophlebitis. Their main disadvantage is the potential hazard to patients with arterial occlusive disease. The application of bandages is dependent on the skill of the practitioner, with experienced clinicians able to consistently apply bandages with pressure ranging from 25–50 mmHg. The less experienced typically achieve pressures in a broader range, from 15–70 mmHg, and deviation on the high end can lead to arterial occlusion in those with pre-existing arterial disease. Therefore, before application, arterial flow should be evaluated by checking the ankle/brachial index, and patients should be instructed on how to properly superimpose each successive layer. After being washed, the bandages tend to lose some of their compressive capability.

Multilayer bandages

Multilayer bandages are a compromise between inelastic bandages and long-stretch elastic bandages. They are often comprised of four super-imposing layers: (1) wool padding for comfort and to absorb exudates; (2) cotton bandage to hold the wool in place; (3) long-stretch elastic bandage for active compression; and finally, (4) cohesive medium-stretch bandages. Significantly, the different indications for the various bandage options are not absolute as the ultimate physiologic effect can be modified by the clinician applying the bandage. Comparative studies assessing the utility of particular bandages for select indications are still inconclusive.

Compression Stockings

Stockings provide an alternative to bandages. Varying in length and by degree of compression, stockings can be used for prophylaxis against DVT or development of varicose veins. Stockings are also indicated after surgery, phlebectomy, or sclerotherapy. Compression following sclerotherapy of varicose veins and larger reticular veins is a universally accepted intervention that encourages the direct apposition of the vein walls so as to decrease the likelihood of thrombus formation and subsequent recanalization of the treated vessel. The avoidance of thrombus formation also appears to limit hyperpigmentation and thrombophlebitis and subsequent telangiectatic matting. However, the utility of stockings following treatment of small telangiectasias contin-ues to be debated. After leg surgery or phlebectomy, stockings help prevent hematomas. During pregnancy, stockings forestall the devel-opment of varicose veins that would otherwise proliferate further due to increased venous pressure and hormonal influences. Pressure stockings are also a key element in the treatment of superficial thrombophlebitis.

There are four stocking compression classes, designated 0 to III (Table 4.3). In each class, there are available various lengths, ranging from socks, to thigh-high, to full-length pantyhose. Proper selection is

Classes of compression stockings		
Compression class	**Pressure (mmHg)**	**Common indications**
0	10–20	Mild functional venous insufficiency
I	20–30	Chronic venous insufficiency, symptomatic varicose veins, DVT
II	30–40	Symptomatic varicose veins, DVT, venous ulcers
III	40–50	Venous ulcers

Table 4.3 Classes of compression stockings

contingent on the indication and the patient's ability to tolerate compression. Elderly patients may have difficulty putting on the stockings, especially the high-compression stockings, and devices have been developed to assist these individuals. An alternative strategy is to superimpose two pairs of compression stockings, with, for example, two pairs of Class 0 stockings offering the same pressure as one pair of Class I stockings. The two separate stockings are easier to pull on. Stockings tend to lose pressure with routine use and washing, and may need to be replaced every 6 months.

Class 0 stockings are indicated in mild functional venous insufficiency that results in minimal varicose veins with associated mild edema or leg fatigue. Chronic venous insufficiency and more severely symptomatic varicose veins should be treated with either Class I or II stockings. Class I or II stockings are also indicated in the outpatient management of DVT as they relieve pain and edema, and enhance thrombus adhesion. Leg ulcer treatment requires Class II or III stockings in addition to local skin treatment. Alternatively, ulcerations may be amenable to other types of compression treatment such as multilayer bandages or inelastic bandages.

There is no consensus on the duration or degree of compression needed after surgery. Although one study has shown equal efficacy between high and low pressure compression stockings in minimizing incidence of bruising and thrombophlebitis after varicose vein surgery, high compression stockings are clearly necessary after sclerotherapy. However, there appears to be no difference between Class I and Class II compression stockings in controlling the objective and subjective parameters of venous insufficiency. Weiss et al studied the duration of compression after sclerotherapy and found that subjects with the most improvement used 3 weeks of compression, followed by the group with 1 week of compression, followed by the group who only used compression for 3 days. All treatment groups had significant improvement compared to the control group that did not receive compression. The 1-week and 3-week groups also experienced less sclerotherapy-associated hyperpigmentation than the 3-day group and the control group.

Treatment of Small Vessel Disease

When larger truncal varicose veins are present, the associated telangiectasias cannot be successfully treated without addressing the underlying hydrostatic pressure elevation. In cases of greater saphenous vein (GSV) incompetence, surgical techniques or endovenous ablative techniques may be required. Ambulatory phlebectomy allows treatment of virtually all large varicose veins while sclerotherapy can be used to treat large varicose veins and reticular varicose veins. Only after the reticular, varicose, and deep incompetent veins have been treated should attention turn to treating the superficial telangiectasias with sclerotherapy or with laser- or light-based devices. In patients with only isolated telangiectasias without pressure problems in larger vessels, sclerotherapy or laser/light therapy may be used primarily (Fig. 4.3).

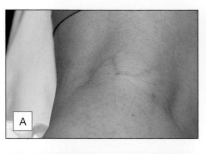
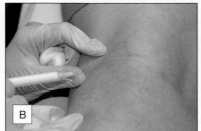
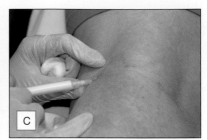
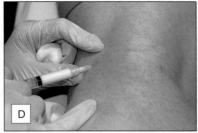
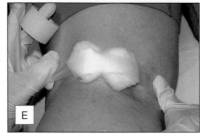

Fig. 4.3 (A) Visualization of the leg vein. **(B)** Two-point counterpressure applied to the injection site. **(C)** Placement of the needle into the vein at 30 degrees. **(D)** Steady injection producing immediate blanching of vessel. **(E)** Immediate application of cotton ball and tape

Sclerotherapy

The goal of sclerotherapy is to intravascularly infuse a chemical irritant to cause irreversible endothelial cellular destruction, which leads to vascular fibrosis and obliteration. Virtually any foreign substance can be utilized to induce venous endothelial damage, and several sclerosing solutions are commercially available for this purpose (Table 4.4). The selection of solution type, concentration, and quantity is dictated by the type and site of the varicosity (Fig. 4.4).

Common sclerosing agents				
Solution	**Category**	**Advantages**	**Disadvantages**	**Brands**
Sodium tetradecyl sulfate	Detergent	Painful only with extravasation; capable of sclerosing larger veins; FDA approved	Necrosis if extravasation >0.25%; pigmentation, matting	Sotradecol (Bioniche Life Sciences Inc., Ontario, Canada) Fibrovein (STD Pharmaceuticals Inc. Hereford, UK)
Polidocanol	Detergent	Always painless; rare necrosis	Urticaria at injection site; no pain to warn of; arteriolar injection; not FDA approved	Aethoxysklerol Kreussler Pharma, Germany
Hypertonic Saline	Hyperosmolar solution	Nonallergenic;	FDA: off-label; painful injections, necrosis, pigmentation, matting	None
Chromated Glycerin	Toxin	Rare matting, pigmentation, necrosis	Too weak for large veins; more viscous; possible allergy; not FDA approved	Scleremo, Lab. Therica, France

Table 4.4 Common sclerosing agents

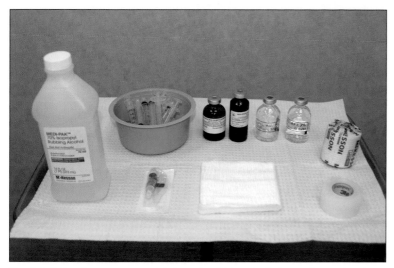

Fig. 4.4 Sclerotherapy tray consisting of: rubbing alcohol, needles and syringes, various sclerosants (shown here-chromated glycerin, 3% sodium tetradecyl sulfate, 0.5% sodium tetradecyl sulfate, and 0.1% sodium tetradecyl sulfate), compression bandage, three-way stopcock, gauze, tape. Not shown are cotton balls

Post-sclerotherapy compression

To decrease the incidence of thrombus formation, which may lead to subsequent recanalization and post-sclerosis pigmentation, compression is also an essential adjunct to sclerotherapy of large varicose veins. Direct apposition of vein walls due to external compression increases the duration of sclerosant contact with the endothelium, thus making the procedure more effective. Lastly, the reduced thrombotic and subsequent inflammatory phlebitic events may also minimize telangiectatic matting. Some authors argue that telangiectasias < 1 mm requires no compression after injection, but there is general agreement that sclerotherapy of larger telangiectasias, venulectasia, reticular veins, and varicose veins must be followed by several days of compression therapy. During sclerotherapy, elastic bandages are commonly applied immediately after the last sclerosant injections. Cotton balls or rubber cushions may be placed under these bandages to provide additional pressure at points of reflux or over larger veins so as to prevent thrombosis. Since the bandages gradually lose the compressive force as they are loosened with patient movement, many clinicians will substitute stockings for bandages after sclerotherapy, or they will advise patients to replace the bandages with stockings in a few hours.

Patient selection

Before embarking on sclerotherapy, a pertinent medical history should be obtained. Specifically, history of lower extremity infections, diabetes, anaphylaxis, and severe asthma should be elicited. Coagulopathies, pregnancy, history of recurrent DVT, and inability to ambulate are contraindications for sclerotherapy. Laboratory tests are usually not necessary except when hypercoagulable states are suspected.

Diagnostic studies such as duplex scanning should be reserved for patients with symptomatic varicosities, varicose veins larger than 4 mm in diameter, or large numbers of spider telangiectasias that are collectively indicative of venous hypertension.

Prior to treatment, patients must understand the procedure and its limitations (Boxes 4.3 and 4.4). The patient must be told that 'perfect legs' are not possible, although significant cosmetic improvement is likely. The physician must never promise complete clearance of all the telangiectasias, and clarify that in the best case, 3–6 treatments may provide about 80% improvement. Treated veins may recur, and new telangiectasias may appear in the future as well. Photographs are useful for both the physician and the patient to document the progress of the treatment. Photographs not only define the pre-treatment extent and the locations of varicose, reticular and telangiectatic veins, but they also document pre-existing scarring or pigmentation.

Lasers and light sources

Lasers have been used to treat leg veins since the 1970s, although laser surgeons did not achieve acceptable results until the advent of the pulsed-dye laser in the 1980s. In the 1990s, the development of lasers with longer wavelengths and longer pulse duration led to improved safety and efficacy, thus creating a niche for lasers in the treatment of leg veins. Like most other lasers for cutaneous indications, lasers used to treat leg veins rely on the principle of selective photothermolysis. The ideal laser must have the following characteristics: (1) a wavelength that is better absorbed by hemoglobin than the surrounding tissue targets (i.e. chromophores); (2) penetration to the depth of the target blood vessel; (3) sufficient energy to damage the blood vessel without injuring the epidermis; and (4) a pulse duration sufficient to slowly coagulate the vessel without damaging the surrounding tissue.

Parameter selection

The challenge in laser treatment of leg veins is that the veins vary widely in size and depth in the skin. Furthermore, the superficial vessels are connected to deeper reticular veins, which often require adjunctive treatment such as sclerotherapy. The choice of wavelength and pulse duration is related to the type and size of the vessels treated. In general, longer wavelengths allow for deeper penetration, and longer pulse durations are needed to slowly heat vessels with larger diameters. Larger spot sizes are associated with reduced skin reflectance and improved laser energy penetrance, resulting in greater effective fluence delivery to the target (Figs 4.5 and 4.6).

Laser selection

Potassium titanyl phosphate (KTP) lasers. The earliest successful treatment of leg veins utilized pulsed lasers and light sources. Pulsed KTP, a 532 nm device, was initially favored because the emitted wavelength was well absorbed by hemoglobin and the KTP crystal in

Expected and minor sequelae of sclerotherapy
■ Hyperpigmentation ■ Edema ■ Matting ■ Pain with injection ■ Localized urticaria ■ Vasovagal reaction ■ Thrombophlebitis ■ Recurrence of treated vessels

Box 4.3 Expected and minor sequelae of sclerotherapy

Rare and serious complications from sclerotherapy
■ DVT ■ Cutaneous necrosis ■ Anaphylaxis ■ Pulmonary emboli ■ Nerve damage

Box 4.4 Rare and serious complications from sclerotherapy

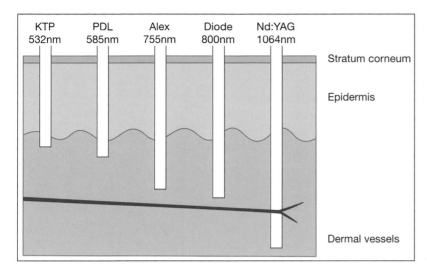

Fig. 4.5 Longer wavelength allows for deeper penetration

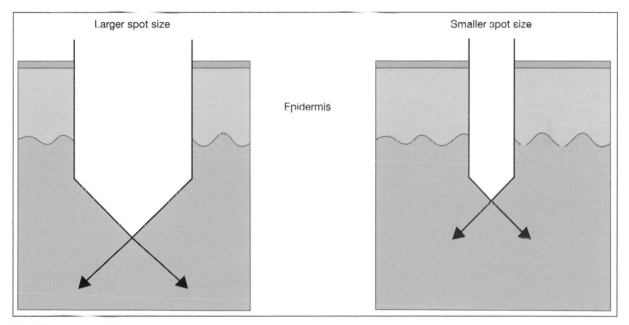

Fig. 4.6 Larger spot size improves penetrance

the laser hardware was reliable and inexpensive. Although millisecond-domain KTP devices proved valuable in treating facial telangiectasias, early experiences with small spot sizes and pulse durations of 10 ms or less were disappointing. Outcomes were much more favorable with the advent of larger spot sizes of 3–5 mm, and longer pulse durations of 10–50 ms at fluences of 12–20 J/cm^2.

The disadvantages of the KTP laser include the fact that thick leg skin can pose a barrier to its limited penetrance, and that the 532 nm wavelength is also heavily absorbed by melanin. Consequently, patients with darker or tanned skin are at high risk of dyspigmentation. Cooling is especially important in these cases to protect the epidermis. Given these limitations, the pulsed KTP is best suited for small, superficial telangiectasias in patients with skin types I–III. Treatment is technique dependent, with multiple passes often needed to achieve the clinical endpoints of vessel spasm or intravascular coagulation, which are associated with better results. However, pulse stacking, or delivering repeated laser pulses to the same site without pause, should be avoided, as this may lead to 'grooving' or scarring.

Pulsed-dye laser. The original pulsed-dye laser (PDL) at 585 nm and 450 µs pulse duration was successful in treating port wine stains, which are composed of very superficial (average depth of 0.46 mm) and minute (100 µm diameter) vessels, usually on the head and neck. However, PDL initially proved to be unsatisfactory in treating leg veins since the short pulse duration was ineffective for deeper and thicker vessels. Given the implications of the theory of selective photo-thermolysis, the ideal pulse duration for destruction of leg veins 0.1 mm to several millimeters in diameter is in the range 1–50 ms. High energy needs to be delivered in a short interval to induce rupture of the vessels with purpura and hemosiderin deposition, seen clinically as long-term hyperpigmentation. The advent of long pulsed-dye laser in the late 1990s enabled treatment of this type. Currently, several devices using rhodamine dye (Cynosure, Berkshire, UK: Photogenica, V-Star; Candela, Wayland, MA: V-Beam) are capable of pulse dura-tions ranging from 1.5–40 ms and wavelengths from 585–600 nm, with the longer wavelengths permitting better penetration to deeper vessels. However, even at these longer PDL wavelengths, melanin absorption is still significant and there is a significant risk of postinflammatory hyperpigmentation if epidermal cooling is insufficient.

Long-pulsed Alexandrite laser. Several other pulsed lasers have successfully exploited the small peak of hemoglobin absorption in the 700–900 nm range. Specifically, the long-pulsed alexandrite, diode, and Nd:YAG lasers are able to treat larger caliber veins; concurrently, their longer wavelengths permit them to penetrate deeper into skin with relatively low levels of absorption by melanin. For example, the 755 nm Alexandrite laser is capable of penetrating 2–3 mm into the skin. Firing with pulse durations of up to 20 ms, this laser can treat small- to medium-diameter vessels with some success.

Diode lasers. Emitting at 800–930 nm, the diode lasers are similar to Alexandrite lasers in their ability to penetrate deeper and target larger reticular veins, and to match the tertiary hemoglobin absorption peak at approximately 900 nm while being absorbed relatively less intensely by melanin.

Long-pulsed Nd:YAG 1064 nm laser. The development of long-pulsed Nd:YAG lasers was an exciting milestone in the treatment of leg veins. The 1064 nm wavelength, longer than the alexandrite and diode, affords even deeper penetration into the skin to target deep, relatively large-caliber vessels. The Nd:YAG laser has a maximum penetration depth of 3 mm, which makes it ideal for destruction of large vessels in the mid-dermis. The scant absorption by melanin also decreases the potential for epidermal damage, even in those with darker skin types. However, the high fluence needed for deep penetration increases the risk for collateral damage as heat is dissipated to the tissue surrounding the target vessels. Furthermore, treatment with the long-pulsed 1064 nm laser is relatively painful (Table 4.5, requiring vigorous epidermal cooling and topical anesthesia. Whereas a complete treatment with other lasers may entail several passes at lower fluences, multiple passes with the high-fluence Nd:YAG laser should be performed with extreme caution. Larger-caliber vessels with diameters of 0.5–3 mm respond best. As with other lasers, the treatment goal is to achieve blanching of the vessels without burning the overlying skin).

Intense pulsed light

The intense pulsed light (IPL) device is typically a noncoherent, 515–1200 nm, flashlamp pumped light source (Palomar, Burlington, MA: Estelux, Medilux; Syneron, Ontario, Canada: Aurora, Polaris; Lumenis, Santa Clara, CA: Quantum, VascuLight). Unique to IPL is the ability to use filters to remove shorter wavelengths in order to increase selectivity. Multiple low-pass filters, rated from 560–755 nm, can be used in this manner. Most useful for vascular lesions are 550 and 570 nm filters that deliver primarily the yellow and red wavelengths with some infrared irradiation.

Broadband IPL takes advantage of the dynamic optical properties of hemoglobin. As vessel size increases from 0.1 mm to 1 mm, and depth increases from 0.3 mm to 1 mm, the peak absorption of hemoglobin shifts from 600 nm to approximately 900 nm. Therefore, a broadband source of 515–1200 nm allows the physician to target the smaller, superficial vessels and the larger, deeper vessels simultaneously. Another practical advantage of the IPL is the relatively larger spot size that facilitates treatment (Fig. 4.7).

Treatment characteristics for Nd:YAG and Alexandrite lasers		
	Nd:YAG	**Alexandrite**
Depth of penetration	⇑	⇓
Hyperpigmentation	⇓	⇑
Pain	⇑	⇓

Table 4.5 Treatment characteristics for Nd:YAG and Alexandrite lasers

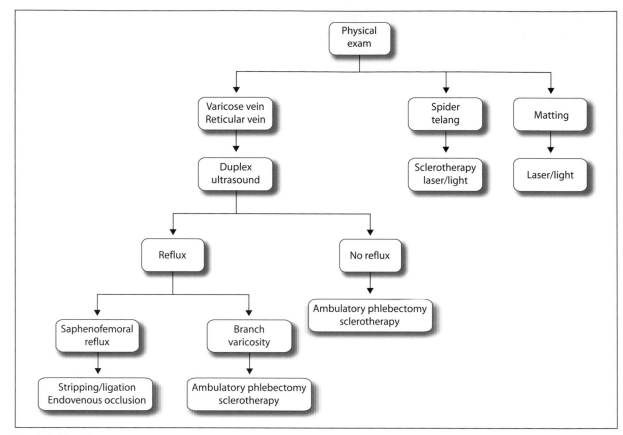

Fig. 4.7 Algorithm to diagnosis and treatment of leg veins

Patient selection

Surgical interventions, endovenous ablative techniques, and sclerotherapy remain the primary choices for varicose veins and reticular veins 3 mm or larger. Lasers and light sources can be considered when telangiectasias 3 mm or smaller are present. Patients best suited for treatment with light-based devices are those: (1) in whom sclerosants are medically contraindicated; (2) who are needle-phobic; (3) who have failed sclerotherapy; (4) whose vessels are too small for cannulation (less than 0.3 mm in diameter); and (5) with foot or ankle vessels that are difficult to treat with sclerotherapy. Since sclerotherapy is heavily technique dependent, physicians who are unfamiliar with sclerotherapy may find more use for lasers. If sclerotherapy is undertaken, treatment should be from largest- to smallest-caliber vessels, starting with varicosities, incompetent perforators, reticular veins, and finally, ending with fine telangiectasias.

Patients should also understand that treatment of leg veins does not culminate in instant improvement. For laser and light devices, 8–12 weeks may be the optimal interval between treatments. Often telangiectasias will ultimately improve despite no signs of change within the initial 2 weeks.

A primary indication for lasers and light sources is telangiectatic matting. Matting refers to multiple tiny new telangiectasias that appear in patients, often after sclerotherapy. Usually matting presents as a confluent, clustered patch of numerous vessels less than 0.2 mm in diameter at the site of treatment. The incidence of matting after sclerotherapy is between 15% and 24%, and although it usually resolves spontaneously in 3–12 months, it can lead to dissatisfaction if patients are not counseled appropriately of the risk before treatment.

Treatment of Large Nontruncal Varicose Veins

All varicosities result from excessive hemodynamic pressure. To correct the problem, sources of high pressure must be eliminated. Even though more distal and smaller veins may be more cosmetically bothersome for the patient, proximal high reflux points must be treated first to prevent immediate recanalization of the finer vessels.

Sclerotherapy

The clinician should adhere to several principles in the sclerotherapy of large varicose veins (Box 4.5). Sclerotherapy can be effective for veins of any size, but the larger the vein, and the higher the pressure at the point of injection, the more the treatments and the higher the concentrations that will be necessary, and the greater the likelihood of recurrence. Even the sclerotherapy of saphenofemoral junction reflux is possible, although the high concentration of injectant required and the need for intraoperative ultrasound guidance may preclude treatment by the novice clinician.

The clinician must remain mindful of the maximum dosage of sclerosant when injecting large veins (Table 4.6).

Foam sclerotherapy

In 1993, Dr Juan Cabrera began using a microfoam preparation of sodium tetradecyl sulfate and polidocanol for sclerotherapy. This represented a revolution in the treatment of venous diseases. The

Steps in the sclerotherapy of large veins
■ Identify and treat reflux points
■ Treat larger veins before smaller veins
■ Treat proximal before distal veins
■ Use maneuvers to empty veins of blood whenever possible
■ Compress immediately

Box 4.5 Steps in the sclerotherapy of large veins

Maximum dosage of sclerosants	
Sclerosant	**Maximum dosage**
Sodium tetradecyl sulfate	10 cc of 3%
Polidocanol	20 cc of 3%
Sclerodex	20 cc per session
Hypertonic 23.4% saline	20 cc per session

Table 4.6 Maximum dosage of sclerosants

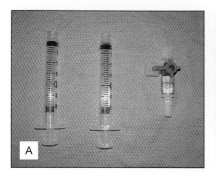
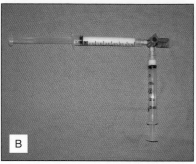
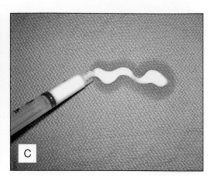

Fig. 4.8 **(A)** Tessari foam technique. Two syringes and a three-way stopcock are needed. One syringe is filled with a detergent sclerosant and the other with air. The two syringes are connected using the stopcock. **(B)** By passing the material quickly back and forth through the stock about 20 times, a foam is produced. **(C)** The foam must be quickly injected before it separates into its air and liquid components

history of foam sclerotherapy actually dates back to Orbach, who in 1944 first proposed the use of foam produced by the simple process of shaking a sclerosant solution in a syringe also containing air. This produced large bubbles with a high air-to-liquid ratio, which proved to be effective for treating smaller veins but not larger veins. Interest faded for several decades, until Cabrera pioneered his newer foam technique. Most recently, Frullini and Tessari have described other variations. The Tessari method, which entails filling one syringe with sclerosant and the other with air, and then passing the material back and forth through a three-way stopcock, is now one of the most widely used techniques due to its simplicity, low cost, and ability to produce high-quality foam. Several large series have been published to document the efficacy and safety of foam sclerotherapy.

Over time, the foam mixture tends to separate into its air and liquid components. The stability of the foam is dependent on the type of sclerosant, concentration of sclerosant, air-to-sclerosant ratio, and duration of mixing. The type of stopcock connector, whether stainless steel, plastic, two way, or three way, appears not to be a significant factor in the quality of the final product (Fig. 4.8).

Advantages of foam

Foam sclerotherapy has several advantages over traditional liquid sclerotherapy. Once a liquid is injected, it mixes with the blood in the vein, thereby diluting the concentration of the sclerosant. Foam, on the other hand, will displace blood, allowing direct contact of the sclerosant with the endothelium. As the efficacy of a given concentration of sclerosant is effectively increased when used as foam instead of liquid, a lower concentration of a given sclerosant can be used. Further, as a fixed volume of liquid can produce up to 4–5 times that volume in foam, a lower total quantity of sclerosant is required when it is delivered as foam. Both of these factors, lower concentrations and decreased quantities of sclerosant, improve the safety of sclerotherapy. Moreover, extravasated foam is much better tolerated than extravasated liquid. Many phlebologists consider yet another advantage of foam to be that the air contained in the foam is echogenic as this dramatically increases visibility and accuracy when performing duplex-guided sclerotherapy.

A 10-year, prospective, controlled randomized trial involving over 800 patients conducted by vascular surgeons in Europe compared six treatment options for varicose veins: (1) liquid sclerotherapy; (2) high-dose liquid sclerotherapy; (3) multiple ligations; (4) stab avulsion; (5) foam sclerotherapy; and (6) ligation followed by sclerotherapy. The report concluded that foam sclerotherapy appears to be more effective than standard dose liquid sclerotherapy, and results can be comparable to surgery. Interestingly, this study also looked at lung scintigraphy in select patients who received foam. The investigators found no perfusion defects even after injections of up to 10 cc of foam. Although foam sclerotherapy is effective for veins of all sizes, some have noted slightly a higher rate of minor side effects, such as pigmentation, inflammation, and minimal necrosis when this method is used to treat small reticular veins and telangiectasias.

Safety concerns

Some uncertainties remain regarding the safety of the foam preparations. The stress that foam places on the human respiratory system is still unclear, although complications rates are exceedingly low. Frullini and Cavezzi proposed a limit of 3 cc of foam per each session of sclerotherapy, although no major complications such as pulmonary embolism, DVT, ischemic lesions, or anaphylactic reactions were recorded. Others suggest less than 10 cc, while some routinely use up to 40 cc without observing serious sequelae. However, when higher doses are used, incidence of dry cough, chest discomfort, transient ischemic attacks, and visual scotomas have been observed.

Ultrasound-guided sclerotherapy

The simplest method of sclerotherapy injection is one based on clinical visualization, without the assistance of localization aids. This is adequate for injection of clearly visible telangiectasias and most reticular veins. However, the injection of deeper varicose veins requires exquisite accuracy, which has led to the introduction of duplex ultrasonography to guide sclerotherapy. Color flow duplex ultrasound has already been immensely helpful in the diagnosis of venous reflux disease and in aiding endovenous radiofrequency and laser ablation techniques. It now enables the experienced clinician to perform sclerotherapy of deeper incompetent vessel or truncal varicosities safely. There are several steps to this process (Box 4.6).

Technique

The procedure begins with preoperative mapping of the areas of superficial reflux. As always, DVT and deep vein incompetence should be ruled out. The areas to be treated are identified, with the ultrasound transducer placed over the introduction site, which should be away

---

Steps in ultrasound-guided sclerotherapy

- Preoperative mapping of area of reflux
- Ultrasound visualization of placement of needle or catheter
- Injection of sclerosant under direct visualization
- Postoperative assessment of result with ultrasound

Box 4.6 Steps in ultrasound-guided sclerotherapy

from important arteries and nerves. The site is first infiltrated with local anesthesia, and the needle is inserted obliquely toward the vessel. The needle should be visualizable on the ultrasound display, and followed as it enters the vessel lumen. The patient should be placed in Trendelenburg position to reduce vessel size, and a syringe should be used to aspirate blood to verify placement. Sclerosant of appropriate concentration and volume for the vessel size can be either directly infused through the needle or through a catheter that can be placed into the vessel via a guidewire. The ultrasound should show the sclerosant flowing into the vessel. The safety of the technique is enhanced when foam is used instead of solution since the echogenicity of foam dramatically increases visibility of the sclerosant and the physician is able to monitor the movement of the sclerosant through the vein. Post-treatment care follows the same protocol as conventional sclerotherapy, with compression and limits on exercise.

The novice phlebologist should be aware that even with ultrasound-guided placement, this technique is not without risk. Inadvertent intra-arterial placement or extravasation can still occur, leading to severe tissue necrosis and nerve injury.

Indications

The advantage of ultrasound-guided sclerotherapy over unaided, or blind, sclerotherapy is visual confirmation of precise placement of the sclerosant. Assisted injection is usually not necessary when the vein is clearly visible from the skin surface, but can be helpful when the vein is obscured. Treating tributaries of the saphenous vein is a particularly strong indication for ultrasound guidance, but other special circumstances may also require this maneuver (Box 4.7).

Doppler-guided sclerotherapy

While duplex ultrasound-guided sclerotherapy has established a new safety standard for sclerotherapy of varicose veins, the cost and operation of a duplex ultrasound device is beyond the capacity of many dermatologists. The introduction of continuous-wave Doppler sclerotherapy in 1992 has made available a more simple and cost-effective variation of the procedure.

Technique

With the patient standing, the varicose vein is first marked by palpation. Once the patient assumes a supine position, additional palpation confirms the absence of a rhythmic arterial bruit, which when present indicates an artery in the area of injection. The Doppler transducer is applied to the marked vein at a 45-degree angle, and with a series of compressions of the vein segment above and below the transducer, the transducer is positioned such that each movement is clearly heard. With the syringe in the other hand, the needle is inserted into the skin 2–3 cm away from the transducer, at a 45-degree angle facing the transducer (Fig. 4.9).

With slight aspiration during needle insertion, the movement of venous blood into the syringe will be audible through the Doppler

---

Indications for DUS-guided sclerotherapy

- Greater saphenous vein without junctional incompetence
- Lesser saphenous vein without junctional incompetence
- Vulvar or scrotal varices
- Varicosities in the obese patient
- Extensive networks of varicosities
- Large incompetent perforating veins

Box 4.7 Indications for DUS-guided sclerotherapy

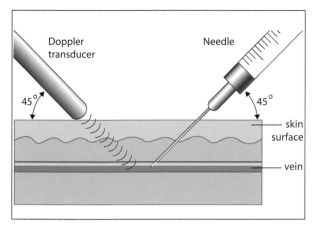

Fig. 4.9 Continuous wave Doppler localizes venous flow at the needle tip. The wave beam and the needle are perpendicular

amplifier once the varicose vein is punctured. Flow into the syringe hub provides visual confirmation. The sclerosant is finally injected, producing a liquid flow sound.

Advantages

Doppler confirmation lowers the risk of extravascular and intra-arterial injections, both of which can lead to necrosis of the skin, or even musculature. The advantage over duplex ultrasound is 2-fold. First, a Doppler transducer is much simpler and faster to operate, and allows the physician to maintain visual contact with the site of injection. Second, the Doppler is much less costly to purchase.

Indications

The indication for Doppler-guided sclerotherapy is based on clinical presentation of the target varicose vein (Table 4.7). When the vein is visible and palpable whether the patient is in a standing or supine

Indications for assisted approaches during sclerotherapy of varicose veins			
Varicose vein	**Unguided**	**Doppler**	**DUS**
Visible and palpable Standing and supine	Yes	Unnecessary	Unnecessary
Palpable standing but not supine	No	Yes	Unnecessary
Impalpable standing or supine	No	No	Yes

Table 4.7 Indications for assisted approaches during sclerotherapy of varicose veins

position, sclerotherapy can proceed with only visual inspection and palpation. But if the vein is palpable with the patient standing but ceases to be palpable once the patient assumes the supine position, the Doppler becomes helpful in guiding the injection. Once the vein is not palpable in either the standing or the supine position, only duplex ultrasound-guided sclerotherapy should be attempted.

Phlebectomy

Phlebectomy is a safe and effective method for removing nearly any incompetent vein below the saphenofemoral and saphenopopliteal junction. The target veins can range from the large truncal veins to their tributaries, perforators, and reticular veins. In experienced hands, a vein can be removed with minimal scarring through an incision as small as 1 mm. Phlebectomy may be employed by itself, or in combination with stripping and ligation, endovenous ablation, or sclerotherapy. The veins most commonly treated by phlebectomy are the accessory saphenous veins of the thigh, pudendal veins, reticular varices in the popliteal folds, reticular veins on the lateral thighs, veins in the ankles, and the dorsal venous networks on the foot.

Technique

Ambulatory phlebectomy requires only a sparse surgical tray. Equipment needed includes a No. 11 blade, an 18 gauge needle, phlebectomy hooks, and mosquito forceps. Physicians vary regarding their preferred phlebectomy hooks, with the most commonly used ones being the Muller, Oesch, Varady, and Ramelet. The various types have different tip sharpness, length and handle size. Most phlebologists use two or more types of different sizes to accommodate veins of varying sizes and depths.

The procedure begins with mapping of the vein and placement of anesthesia along the segment of the vein to be removed. The most common technique is perivenous infiltration using Lidocaine with epinephrine. Recently, tumescent anesthesia, an extremely dilute aqueous solution of Lidocaine with admixed epinephrine and bicarbonate, has gained popularity. Tumescing the area allows for less painful injections, hydrodissection-assisted separation of the vein, intraoperative hemostasis, and persistent local compression via mass effect postoperatively. Once anesthesia is obtained, a small incision with either a No. 11 blade or 18 gauge needle is made over the vein. The stem of the phlebectomy hook is inserted to dissect the vein and loosen it from its fibrous attachments. The hook is then used to grasp and externalize the vein, with this followed by clamping and securing the vein with mosquito forceps. By carefully pulling on the vein with the help of several mosquito forceps, a segment of the vein is removed intact. The physician then repeats this process with more incisions along the course of the vein until the entire length of targeted vein is eliminated.

Postoperatively, the incisions are covered with sterile gauze or absorbent pads, then secured with tape. Compression is applied with long-stretch bandages or compression stockings, and ambulation is encouraged to avoid DVT. The wound dressing may be changed in 24–48 hours, but the compression should continue for at least 7 days.

Although usually more time consuming than sclerotherapy, ambulatory phlebectomy has several advantages, including the avoidance of potential intra-arterial injection, extravasation necrosis, and hyperpigmentation. Finally, unlike with sclerotherapy, only one treatment is needed (Fig. 4.10).

Treatment of Perforating Veins

Perforating veins (PVs) join the superficial and deep veins and channel blood flow from the superficial system to the deep venous system. There are numerous PVs in each leg. Clinically and hemodynamically important PVs are located at four sites: (1) the thigh; (2) upper medial lower leg; (3) lower medial lower leg; and (4) knee. Although no strict criteria exist for the diagnosis of incompetent PVs, most authors

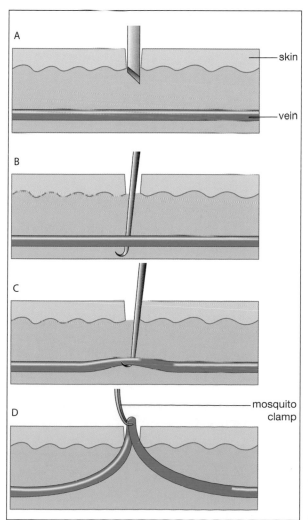

Fig. 4.10 (**A**) Puncture skin with 18 gauge needle or small incision with No. 11 blade. (**B**) Introduction of hook through incision and dissection of tissue around vein with stem of the hook. (**C**) Hooking the vein upward through the incision. (**D**) Grasping and extracting the vein using mosquito clamps

consider reflux of more than 0.5 seconds and relative diameter of the vein as evidence of incompetence.

PVs can be classified into several types. When the PV is primarily insufficient, likely the result of an inherited weakness in the vein wall, direct treatment of the PV can lead to clinical improvement. Likewise, when the incompetent PV is associated with isolated deep venous reflux, direct treatment may reduce symptoms. When a PV becomes incompetent as a result of a proximal superficial venous insufficiency that places hemodynamic pressure on the distal veins, treatment of this proximal superficial reflux should be the first priority. This is the most common cause of incompetent PV. Treatment of the PV when it is acts as a collateral pathway for a deep venous obstruction is contraindicated.

The value of treating a PV alone is difficult to assess. It is difficult to isolate the significance of an incompetent PV in the context of co-existing venous insufficiency. In most cases, an incompetent PV and superficial venous reflux are treated simultaneously to achieve clinical improvement. In fact, whether PVs should be treated at all remains controversial, but once a decision to eliminate incompetent PVs has been made, several techniques are possible (Fig. 4.11).

Subfascial endoscopic perforating surgery

Linton's procedure, described in the 1930s, involves a long skin incision to perform open ligation of the PVs. This procedure has now been largely abandoned due to unacceptable level of morbidity. Instead, subfascial endoscopic perforating surgery (SEPS) is now a widely accepted minimally invasive surgical technique to eliminate incompetent PVs. In SEPS, through a small incision in the upper calf, an endoscope is introduced between the fascia and the underlying muscle. With endoscopic visualization, an instrument is advanced to intercept and eliminate all visible PVs. SEPS is associated with much lower morbidity than the classic Linton procedure, with the former method having wound complication rates ranging from 4–6%. Usually performed in combination with ablation of the superficial venous reflux, SEPS in both short-term and medium-term clinical series has been associated with high rates of healing of venous ulcerations and low recurrence rates compared to compression bandaging alone. However, the very long-term benefits and effects of SEPS are not yet known.

Sclerotherapy

The role of sclerotherapy in the treatment of incompetent PVs has yet to be defined. Only a few studies have attempted to characterize the efficacy of sclerotherapy, and using various techniques and sclerosants, rates of successful occlusion ranging from 20–90% have been reported. Sclerotherapy of perforating veins carries higher risk than sclerotherapy of smaller telangiectasias since perforating arteries often accompany perforating veins. Inadvertent injection into arteries can lead to significant tissue necrosis, with the further possibility of the sclerosant flowing into the deep venous system, causing DVT. Other complica-

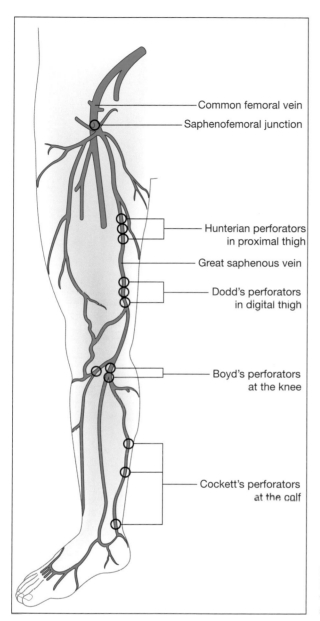

Fig. 4.11 Greater saphenous vein as it branches from the common femoral vein. The principal perforators are shown

- Common femoral vein
- Saphenofemoral junction
- Hunterian perforators in proximal thigh
- Great saphenous vein
- Dodd's perforators in digital thigh
- Boyd's perforators at the knee
- Cockett's perforators at the calf

tions of sclerotherapy of incompetent PVs, including hyperpigmentation, matting, and phlebitis, are similar to those of sclerotherapy elsewhere. To minimize arterial cannulation and subsequent ulceration during sclerotherapy of PVs, ultrasound guidance may be enlisted.

Treatment of Truncal Incompetence

Sclerotherapy

Sclerotherapy of truncal veins (greater saphenous vein or lesser saphenous vein) or their tributaries may be attempted with concentrated sclerosant. To ensure maximal contact of the sclerosant and the endothelium, and to reduce the dilutional effect that occurs when sclerosant mixes with blood, the physician may reduce the volume of the blood in the veins to be injected by placing the patient in a supine or Trendelenburg position, or by elevating the leg.

Examination of the treated veins can be performed 2 weeks following the injection. If closure has not been achieved, treatment can be repeated.

Stripping and ligation

Although recent advancements have allowed for minimally invasive techniques, such as endovenous ablation techniques or ultrasound-guided sclerotherapy, for eliminating truncal reflux, conventional surgical techniques are still useful in many instances. On the one hand, the oldest surgical approaches, such as the Linton technique, have been abandoned due to unacceptable complication rates, and prior to the advent of readily available duplex ultrasound, incorrect diagnosis often led to incomplete treatment or stripping of the wrong vein, with a subsequent high rate of recurrences. However, modern open surgical approaches offer dramatically reduced complication rates and recovery time, with an acceptable cosmetic outcome.

The modern perforate-invaginate (PIN) technique starts with ligation of the saphenofemoral junction and its tributaries through a 2–3 cm incision in the groin. The greater saphenous vein is then removed through this incision with the help of a stripping tool that consists of a modified wire, which is threaded through the GSV to the level of the upper calf, where it is externalized. At this point, an acorn-shaped head is attached to the proximal end of the stripper wire. As the wire is pulled out in the distal direction, the vein invaginates into itself, as it is pulled the entire length. The lesser saphenous vein may be treated by the same method, but this carries a high risk of nerve injury.

High ligation of the saphenofemoral junction without concurrent saphenoectomy is associated with a high rate of recurrence. Accessory veins, collateral veins, and tributaries can dilate rapidly and re-establish the pattern of reflux. Ligation of distal varicosities alone, as taught in vascular surgery programs in the 1970s and 1980s, is also inadequate because the origin of reflux in the saphenous trunk remains unaddressed, and the point of high hemodynamic pressure persists. Unsatisfied patients tend to return with recurrent varicosities.

The invasive nature of vein surgery still carries risk for various complications (Box 4.8). The most serious complications is DVT, leading to pulmonary embolism. To avoid this potentially fatal outcome, postoperative compression and ambulation is mandatory. Other undesired effects are hematoma and wound infection, the incidence of which can be minimized by good surgical technique. Inadvertent injury to the sural and saphenous nerve can occur, and tends to be very disconcerting to patients. Although annoying, telangiectatic matting and hyperpigmentation are usually temporary and amenable to treatment.

Potential complications from vein surgery

Common complications
- Scarring
- Thrombophlebitis
- Hyperpigmentation
- Telangiectatic matting

Rare and/or serious complications
- DVT
- Pulmonary embolism
- Nerve injury
- Postoperative wound infection

Box 4.8 Potential complications from vein surgery

Endovenous ablation

Successful long-term treatment of truncal varicose veins requires the elimination of both the highest point of reflux and elimination of the incompetent venous segment. Until recent years, the standard for treatment of saphenous vein reflux has been ligation with or without stripping, despite little evidence of long-term success with ligation alone. Recurrences occur due to re-anastamoses of previously ligated tributaries or failure to ligate a functional tributary, which subsequently becomes varicose. Furthermore, the traditional method of stripping involves significant scars and a long, painful recovery period. Sclerotherapy of truncal varicosities under ultrasound guidance is an alternative, but an imperfect one, with a 10–42% risk of recanalization within 1 year. With foam sclerotherapy, the long-term success rate may increase, but the safety of the procedure is a consideration, as the sclerosant may flow into the deep venous system.

A relatively recent technological innovation involves endovenous occlusion with radiofrequency (RF) energy. Under duplex ultrasound guidance, an RF catheter is inserted into the greater saphenous vein (GSV) and positioned at the base of the terminal valve. The RF energy is then delivered while the catheter is slowly withdrawn. This process enables shrinkage of the vein wall without electrocoagulation of blood. At the conclusion of the procedure, there is no flow through the greater saphenous vein. Over time, patient symptoms improve and distal varicosities shrink. Short-term advantages of the RF procedure over traditional stripping and ligation have been documented in prospective multi-center randomized comparisons. In general, advantages of endovascular obliteration of the GSV over conventional vein stripping include a diminution of pain and shorter recovery time. Long-term persistence of results has been quite favorable as well, with 2-year follow-up results confirming elimination of GSV reflux in more than 90% of treated limbs, with symptomatic improvement in 95% of limbs.

Alternatively, endovenous ablation can employ laser sources, with the naked laser fiber inserted into the GSV and extracted during the laser-on period in the same manner as with RF. Unlike RF ablation, laser ablation uses optically generated thermal energy rather than radiofrequency-derived thermal energy to damage the vein wall. In a study by Min et al, over 400 varicose veins were successfully treated over a 3-year period with 810 nm diode laser energy delivered directly into the GSV. Long-term results in patients treated with endovenous lasers demonstrate a recurrence rate of less than 7% at 2-year follow up. A single early study using the animal model suggests that the 810 nm endovenous laser technique may be at a higher risk compared to the RF technique for vein perforations and may occasionally fail to cause significant collagen shrinkage, which in theory may lead to early recanalization and risk of recurrence; however, more recent human data has not revealed such a risk of recurrence. Physician experience with endovenous laser ablation continues to increase, and the available evidence indicates that the procedure is a safe and effective technique in the same general category as RF ablation. The increased use of the

1320 nm Nd:YAG for laser ablation promises to make this procedure even more well tolerated and effective.

Integrating Therapeutic Options

Treating varicosities successfully requires rational selection of interventions (Fig. 4.7). To choose the optimal therapeutic technique, physicians must first diagnose the origin of the reflux. Physical examination is necessary to determine whether the surface telangiectasias originate from a deeper source of incompetence. To make this determination, it is necessary to have adequate knowledge of the superficial venous anatomy and possess the proper diagnostic tools and equipment, including ultrasound devices. If present, reticular or larger varicose veins should be eliminated first either surgically or through endovenous ablation. This should be followed by sclerotherapy of the remaining vessels, from largest to smallest. Vessels that do not respond to sclerotherapy, that are too small to be injected, or that remain after sclerotherapy, should be considered for laser and light treatment. A primary indication for laser and light sources is telangiectatic matting (Fig. 4.7).

Further Reading

Breu FX, Guggenbichler S 2004 European Consensus Meeting on Foam Sclerotherapy. Dermatologic Surgery 30:709–17

Cornu-Thenard A, de Cottreau H, Weiss RA 1995 Continuous wave Doppler-guided injections. Dermatologic Surgery 21:867–870

Hsu TS, Weiss RA 2003 Foam sclerotherapy: a new era. Archives of Dermatology 139:1494–1496

Min RJ, Khilnani N, Zimmet SE 2003 Endovenous laser treatment of saphenous vein reflux: long-term results. Journal of Vascular Interventional Radiology 14:991–996

Ramelet AA 2002 Compression therapy. Dermatologic Surgery 28:6–10

Ramelet AA 2002 Phlebectomy. Technique, indications and complications. International Angiology 21(Suppl 1):46–51

Rao J, Goldman MP 2005 Stability of foam in sclerotherapy: differences between sodium tetradecyl sulfate and polidocanol and the type of connector used in the double-syringe system technique. Dermatologic Surgery 31:19–22

van Neer PA, Veraart JC, Neumann HA 2003 Venae perforantes: a clinical review. Dermatologic Surgery 29:931–942

Weiss RA, Feied CF, Weiss MA 2001 Vein diagnosis & treatment: A comprehensive approach. McGraw-Hill

Weiss RA, Sadick NS, Goldman MP, Weiss MA 1999 Post-sclerotherapy compression: controlled comparative study of duration of compression and its effects on clinical outcome. Dermatologic Surgery 25:105–108

Sclerotherapy

5

David M. Duffy

Introduction

The object of this chapter is to enable the reader to recognize a variety of clinically observable features that underlie the occurrence of successful or unsuccessful results following sclerotherapy. For the sake of brevity, a number of the strategies and concepts that have evolved and proved useful in the treatment of thousands of patients over a 26-year period will be presented in bullet, table, or question and answer format. For many dermatologists, telangiectasias and small reticular veins unassociated with significant venous disease will be present in most of the patients who request treatment. Accordingly, the preponderance of information presented here will deal with small vessel sclerotherapy.

Variability

Sclerotherapy is an art and not a science. Any modality that destroys tissue can produce a wide and often unpredictable range of responses. Indeed, patient response to venous trauma via sclerotherapy, electronic (lasers etc.), or surgery can vary enormously from person to person. It's also worth remembering that when treating any individual, outcomes can be affected by multiple variables including anatomical location, intrinsic vessel fragility, and important connections between visible veins and the deeper venous circulation. These connections may result in far different treatment outcomes when treating one leg vs. the other. Unexplained innate variability and lack of understanding about the multiple factors that affect it, has provoked a great deal of controversy regarding the 'ideal way' to treat unwanted veins. Personal experience, confirmed by review of tens of thousands of before and after photographs, suggests that:

- There is no cure for varicose or spider veins, and good or bad results can occur using any treatment protocol
- What happens in the short term often changes in the long run
- No single treatment 'recipe' will consistently produce optimum results
- Of all the identifiable characteristics that affect treatment outcomes, vessel size is the best prognosticator of treatment effects and the occurrence of common complications (Fig. 5.1)

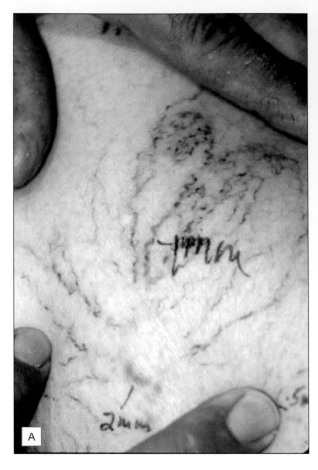

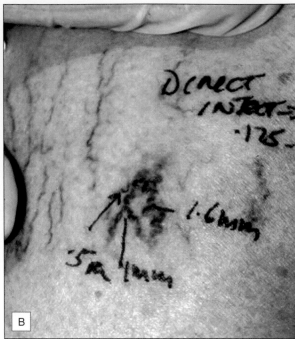

Fig. 5.1 (**A** and **B**) Measurements of vessel size reveal typical variability associated with specific vessel sizes

- Treatment of telangiectasias 0.5 mm in diameter and smaller will often provide the greatest range of outcomes and patterns of response as vessels larger than this size usually respond to treatment much more predictably
- Good results can be obtained by injecting telangiectasias directly without treating reticular veins
- Reticular veins can be destroyed with pigmentation/matting, sometimes leaving telangiectasias unaffected (Fig. 5.2).

Divide and Conquer

Sclerotherapy is best divided into two components, the first being large-vessel sclerotherapy, which treats refluxing axial varicosities (saphenofemoral and saphenopopliteal junctions), nonsaphenous truncal varicosities, perforators and large (> 3 mm in diameter) reticular veins. Traditionally sclerotherapy was considered a poor second to surgical intervention for the treatment of junctional reflux and vessels > 8 mm in diameter. However, significant advances in sclerotherapy, such as the development of foam sclerosants and imaging techniques (which are

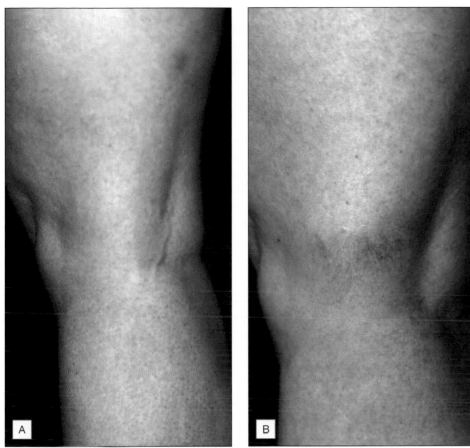

Fig. 5.2 (A) This reticular vein measuring 1.3 mm in diameter was cosmetically unattractive to this patient. **(B)** A post-treatment photograph reveals neovascularization (matting) which was even more unattractive to the patient. Although almost nothing has been published regarding complications following injection of reticular veins, the author has found matting to be a relatively common occurrence in this area

facilitated by the use of foam), have made large vessel treatment more feasible.

Advances in Large Vessel Sclerotherapy: Foam/Imaging Techniques

Foam

The use of foam sclerosing agents for the treatment of large and small varicose veins started as early as 1939. All foam preparations are generally considered to be three to four times more potent than equivalent concentrations and volumes of liquid sclerosants. This increased potency is related to several factors, including an increase in the effective surface area of foams compared with liquid, and the displacement of blood from the treated vein, which produces prolonged undiluted intimal contact.

Foam also produces increased vasospasm and sclerosis of veins at a greater distance from the injection site than can liquid preparations, and can be used in much smaller volumes and concentrations (with presumably less risk of tissue necrosis). Foams are 'dramatically more visible' than liquids on duplex imaging. Foam sclerosants have also proved valuable for the treatment of venous malformations. The downside of foam is the difficulty in using it clinically (i.e. aspiration is difficult), and the fact that extemporaneous preparations of foams are hard to precisely duplicate and given there are to date no standarized foam preparations available. This makes it difficult to establish uniform treatment protocols or compare the efficacy of different types of foam in specific applications. In addition, the United States FDA has not scrutinized, let alone approved, any type of foam for any purpose. Wollmann has extensively detailed both the history and enormous number of variables (e.g. bubble size, uniformity, temperature, sclerosant/gas ratios, type of gas, type of sclerosant etc.) that influence the effect of foam preparations. Although foam sclerotherapy has the potential to revolutionize the treatment of large refluxing veins, it is at this point in time in the early phase of integration into common usage. Under the wrong circumstances, when treating patients with patent ductus arteriosis, a bolus of foam could theoretically lodge in the lungs and produce pulmonary fibrosis. Migraine symptoms, unintended thrombosis of vessels at distant sites, and other complications associated with superpotent sclerosants may be increased using foam sclerotherapy. For large vessels associated with significant reflux, some combination of foam sclerotherapy, surgical intervention, and endovenous laser or radiofrequency devices may be employed synergistically by individuals experienced in their use. Good results following any modality will depend not so much upon the specific treatment employed, but on the expertise of the practitioner.

Duplex problems

Although real-time duplex imaging is an invaluable aid to placing needles in the right position, it is by no means perfect. Duplex scans, after all, are a two-dimensional view of a three-dimensional process. In at least one case, a lawsuit has been filed (unpublished personal communication) when severe tissue necrosis necessitating in the amputation of a lower limb occurred despite the use of duplex guidance during the administration of foam. The concentration of foam in this case may have been much greater than recommended by most authorities.

Personal experience with foam

Over the last several years the author has treated approximately 500 patients presenting with a wide range of vessel diameters using one part polidocanol to three or four parts room air prepared foam using the double-syringe method. The author has found foam preparations are particularly effective for refluxing vessels 4–5 mm in diameter but unnecessarily cumbersome and no more effective than liquid sclerosants for smaller vessels, particularly telangiectasias. Foam takes time to prepare, deteriorates quickly at room temperature, and viscous foams prepared using a higher sclerosant concentration flow more effectively when large-bore needles such as the MaxFlow™ (Richard James, Peabody, MA) are employed. As noted earlier, aspiration is often difficult. Several technique changes must be employed. Compression is often delayed for several minutes following the procedure to avoid extending foam into areas where unintended thrombosis can occur. For this reason, spot compression is not employed. Most importantly, a 10-fold increase in the occurrence of superficial thrombophlebitis has been observed (unpublished personal data) following the use of foam compared with liquids. Ordinarily, patients only require one thrombectomy to evacuate thrombi in treated vessels. However, following use of foam preparations, recurrent thrombi and thrombophlebitis occurring up to 1–2 months after treatment sometimes requires multiple thrombectomies.

Small-vessel Sclerotherapy

Small-vessel sclerotherapy deals with reticular veins < 3 mm in diameter and a wide spectrum of telangiectasias. An important distinction between large refluxing vessels and small vessels is the fact that large vessel treatments are often employed as a medical necessity and are appropriately billed for insurance compensation. Small-vessel sclerotherapy is often, but not always, an elective cosmetic procedure, although telangiectasias and small reticular veins are occasionally symptomatic.

Advances in small-vessel sclerotherapy

Advances in small-vessel sclerotherapy are evolutionary, not revolutionary. Although some authorities have proposed specific guidelines, there are very few absolutes.

Controversies regarding small-vessel sclerotherapy involve the importance of venous reflux and venous hypertension, the need (or lack thereof) to treat large vessels before small, and the importance of compression when treating telangiectasias. Refluxing reticular veins have been implicated as a prime etiologic factor for the development of telangiectasias, although credible arguments against this notion have been presented. Lasers and light sources that need to traverse the skin to reach the vessel, although highly promoted, are expensive, painful, time consuming, and decidedly inferior alternatives to sclerotherapy as the treatment of choice (Figs 5.3, 5.4). Their use should be reserved for patients who are allergic to sclerosants, are needle phobic, have vessels too small for inexperienced phlebologists to cannulate, or are unresponsive to prior sclerotherapy. In contrast, endovenous radiofrequency and laser devices that are used to treat large vessels are a promising new therapy for smaller vessels as well.

Classifying Veins: A New Paradigm

In 1988, presented a classification system for small vessels which included approximate vessel diameters, anatomical features, color, and

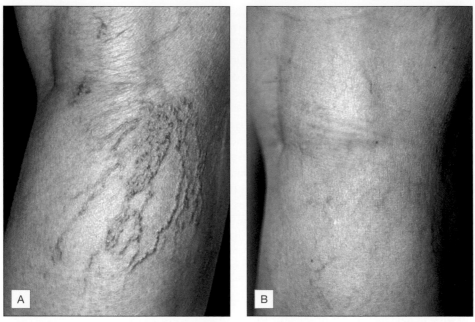

Fig. 5.3 (A and B) These photographs present results obtained following one injection. Sclerotherapy is less painful, faster and less expensive than laser treatments for lower extremity veins

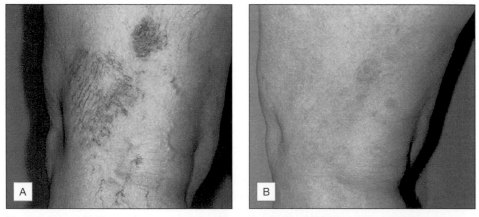

Fig. 5.4 (A and B) These photographs present results obtained following three treatment sessions using both intense pulsed light and the 1064 Nd:YAG laser. In this case, $200,000 dollars worth of electronic gadgetry produced results that could have been duplicated with 25¢ of sclerosing solution and a lot less pain

relationships to the saphenous system. This classification has been modified, expanded and presented by other authors. Although this scheme proved useful for categorizing and optimizing treatment of specific types of vessels, it does not recognize the existence of a large number of identifiable variables that affect the outcome of sclerotherapy nor does it acknowledge the relationship of vessel size to intrinsic patterns of long and short-term responses to sclerotherapy. In addition, it does not address the emergence of a specific class of extremely resistant telangiectasias (usually ≤ 0.2 mm in diameter), which develop after previous sclerotherapy treatments. This process may be part of a persistent longlasting vascular remodeling, which has become the primary cause of patient dissatisfaction following small-vessel sclerotherapy.

Basic Patterns of Response

Following use of any modality, three responses to treatment will be noted, and since most patients present with vessels of various diameters, a mixture of these patterns is usually observed:

1. Gradual fibrosis (fading) in which small telangiectasias gradually fade and fragment, a process usually not associated with pigment or palpable thrombi and occurring following multiple treatments over several months (small vessel pattern) (Fig. 5.5).
2. Rapid, immediate destruction, often associated with pigment and palpable thrombi following treatment of larger, more fragile telangiectasias and varicose veins. This process often occurs within several days of treatment (large-vessel pattern) (Fig. 5.6).
3. Resistance, which occurs following the treatment of varicose veins, is often associated with dilutional factors that must be compensated for by using more concentrated sclerosants. When resistance occurs in very small telangiectasias, the cause is unknown, but since it is rare in patients who have not received previous treatment and extremely common in those who have, it may be due to molecular biological processes such as failure to trigger apoptosis, or a

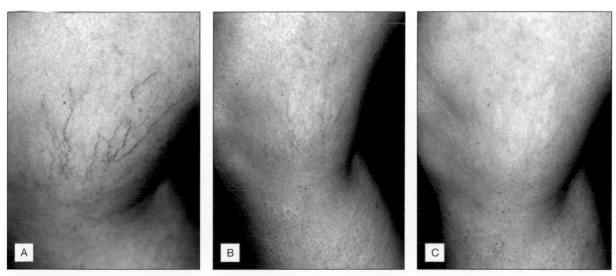

Fig. 5.5 (A) Pretreatment appearance of vessels involving the inner knee, varying in size from 0.1 mm to approximately 0.5 mm in diameter. **(B)** This photograph taken 3 months after two treatments reveals complete disappearance of the large vessels with substantial fading in the smaller ones, a typical pattern. **(C)** This photograph taken 10 months after the second treatment reveals almost complete resolution. The inner knees are an area subject to matting and should be treated cautiously with low concentration of sclerosants

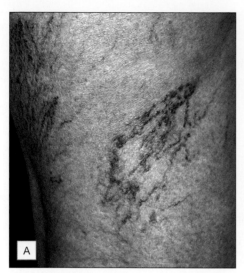 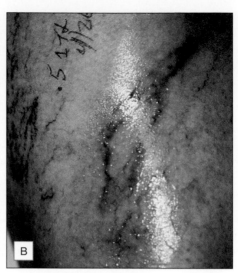

Fig. 5.6 **(A)** These pretreatment photographs reveal fragile, thin-walled, elevated tortuous vessels 0.6–1.0 mm in diameter. **(B)** This photo demonstrates pigmentation, which can occur following low sclerosant concentrations when treating vessels of this type

heightened angiogenic response (accelerated wound healing), as a consequence of previous vascular trauma.

Vessel Size: New Golden Rules

Of all the parameters that affect treatment outcomes, vessel size is by far the most meaningful prognosticator for treatment outcomes. This is not to say that vessels will always respond stereotypically on the basis of vessel size. The concentration of sclerosant necessary to destroy veins varies a great deal from person to person and vessels of the same size will sometimes display similar patterns of response despite wide variations in sclerosant concentration (Figs 5.7–5.9). Given this degree of variability it is more prudent to consider typical patterns rather than make precise predictions. Nevertheless, for telangiectasias $\leq$ 0.5 mm in diameter, very small changes in vessel size can produce fundamental differences in the way vessels respond to treatment and the occurrence of common complications. Although sclerosant concentrations and other factors can alter treatment responses, careful measurement of vessel size will often accurately predict:

- Whether vessels will respond gradually to repeated treatments (usually without associated pigmentation or thrombi)
- Whether vessels will respond rapidly, often in association with thrombi and pigmentation
- The number of treatments necessary
- Whether the vessels will be resistant to treatment.
- How long vessels have been present
- The occurrence of complications (pigment, thrombi, resistance)
- The likelihood of underlying reflux/venous hypertension

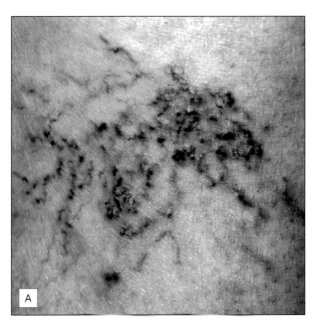
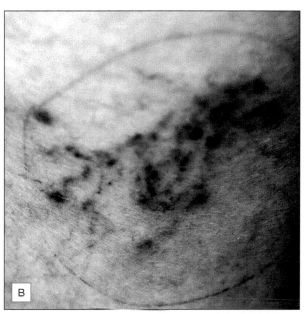

Fig. 5.7 (A) Pretreatment photograph, vessels measured 0.6–1.0 mm in diameter were elevated and tortuous. (B) Results were seen 1 week after one treatment with 0.5% polidocanol

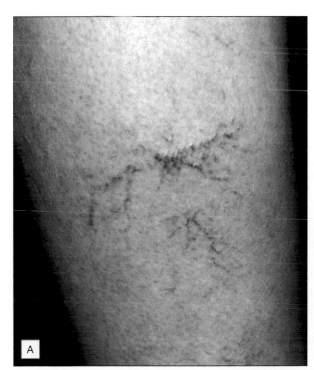
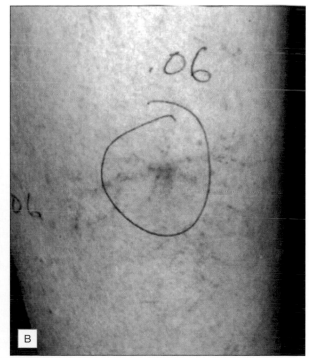

Fig. 5.8 (A) Pretreatment photographs, vessels 0.5–0.8 mm in diameter elevated and tortuous. (B) This post-treatment photograph taken 3 months after two treatments using 0.06% polidocanol produced a more gradual destruction with less thrombosis than a single injection of 0.5%, an 8-fold difference in concentration.

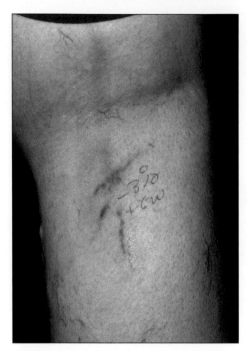

Fig. 5.9 This photograph reveals thrombosis and pigmentation noted 6 weeks after one treatment with 3% polidocanol. Equivalent results can often be obtained using vastly different sclerosant strengths. Accordingly, strategies relating vessel size to sclerosant concentrations are a highly individual affair

- Optimal sclerosant concentrations
- Sensitivity to changes in sclerosant concentration
- The need for compression.

A Word about the Literature and Vessel Size

Phlebology literature at large views all veins between 0.1 mm and 1 mm in diameter as a homogeneous entity. There are at least seven categories of vessels in this size range, each exhibiting more or less typical patterns of response and sensitivity to sclerosants, as well as distinct differences involving a host of other variables. When practitioners attribute optimal results (particularly the number of treatments necessary to destroy the vessel and the occurrence of pigmentation or thrombosis) to some technique strategy, their observations have limited utility unless the specific size of the vessel is duly noted. In truth, very small vessels ($\leq$ 0.3 mm in diameter) routinely require several treatments for eradication, and even when using high concentrations of sclerosants, rapid results, pigmentation, and palpable thrombosis rarely occur. Conversely, veins > 0.4 mm in diameter are routinely eradicated in one treatment, a process often associated with pigmentation and thrombi. Higher sclerosant concentrations will routinely produce more tissue trauma, sometimes resulting in excessive pigmentation, bulky thrombi, and increased neovascularization. There is no foolproof way to determine optimal sclerosant concentrations.

Categorizing Vessels by Size: Effect of Previous Treatments upon Microtelangiectasias

Very small vessels can be divided into two distinct categories on the basis of their response or resistance to sclerotherapy.

1. **Responsive**
   - ▪ **0.1–0.2 mm in diameter**: Previously untreated (virgin) veins in this size range can usually be effectively treated. They often require at least three treatments to induce a slow process of fading, which may involve the body's own genetic machinery to destroy partially damaged cells in the vessel walls (apoptosis). The use of higher concentrations often will not produce faster results and may lead to more matting. Compression does not appear to be of benefit when treating very small vessels. Pigmentation is rare. Treatment is usually carried out at 4–6-week intervals. Resistance is extremely uncommon in previously untreated vessels measuring ≤ 0.2 mm in diameter. Pigmentation is extremely rare for all vessels in this size range (Fig. 5.5).
2. **Resistant telangiectasias (matting/second-generation vessels):**
   - ▪ **0.1–0.2 mm in diameter**: Vessels in this size range which remain or occur after previous treatments, are often refractory to treatment within a given time frame, and are the number one cause of dissatisfaction following small-vessel sclerotherapy (Fig. 5.10).

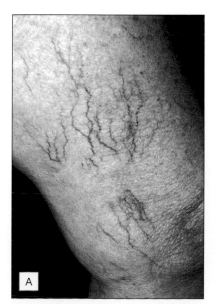 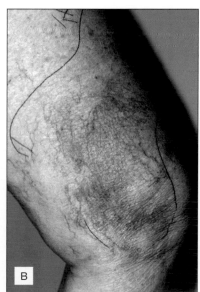 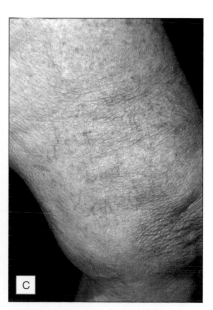

Fig. 5.10 (A) Pretreatment photographs reveal vessels varying in size from 0.2–0.8 mm in diameter. **(B)** This photograph, taken approximately 1 year later reveal extensive neovascularization resistant to several treatments carried out over a 6-month period. **(C)** 1 year later these neovascular vessels had resolved spontaneously. Deferred treatments are often the best way to approach neovascularization (matting)

This type of vasculature is most common on the inner and outer thighs within 25 cm of the knees. The author's experience suggests that vessels of this type are best treated by tincture of time, being treated no more than two to three times yearly. With sufficient time these vessels may resolve spontaneously or become responsive to sclerotherapy and other modalities. It has not been shown that the injection of reticular veins or elimination of reflux are of any particular benefit.

- **0.3–0.5 mm in diameter**: Good news begins at 0.3 mm. These vessels usually require several treatments and fade slowly over several months without pigmentation or thrombi. The usual treatment interval for vessels in this size range is every 4–6 weeks, whether or not the patient has been treated before. As vessels become fractionally larger, a second (large-vessel pattern) supervenes. At 0.4 mm and 0.5 mm in diameter, pattern overlap occurs. Vessels of this size can undergo the small-vessel fading pattern or be destroyed rapidly, a process sometimes associated with pigmentation and thrombosis. About 25% of vessels measuring 0.4 mm and about 50% of those measuring 0.5 mm will respond rapidly. Changes in concentration may affect rapidity of this process. Higher sclerosant concentrations are routinely associated with more rapid results associated with increased thrombosis and pigmentation (Figs 5.8, 5.9). In some cases, injection of reticular veins that are in direct communication with clusters of telangiectasias produce dilutional effects that may reduce hyperpigmentation in fragile veins. This technique also permits fewer needle sticks. In other patients, injecting the reticular veins does not appear to modify outcomes one way or another.

- **0.6–0.9 mm in diameter**: Vessels in this size range are often purple or blue–green in color. They can be extremely fragile and often have been present for many years (Fig. 5.6). Clusters of elevated and tortuous vessels of this size often suggest long-standing venous hypertension or reflux. Their presence should prompt a more thorough evaluation. These vessels usually require only one treatment. It is sometimes beneficial to employ more dilute sclerosants and/or compression to minimize pigmentation and clotting that routinely follows treatment. Sometimes the injection of larger, adjacent reticular veins dilute injected sclerosants and may reduce pigmentation and thrombi when treating fragile, communicating telangiectasias. A constellation of bruising, thrombi, and pigmentation often makes treated veins of this type look worse before they look better. Patients may be reassured using postoperative photographs of patients with similar veins.

- **1–5 mm in diameter**: Large greenish-blue vessels (i.e. the color of the veins on the backs of hands) are usually destroyed in one or two treatments, a process that is often followed by clotting and pigmentation. Vascular fragility is a highly individual matter. Certain individuals will experience rapid destruction of vessels not associated with thrombosis or pigmentation using a wide

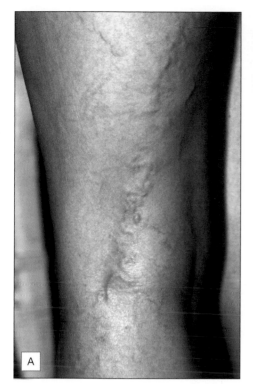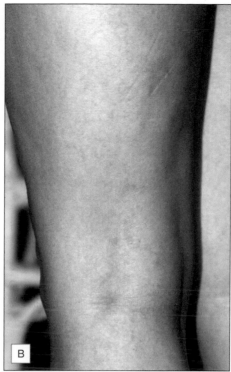

Fig. 5.11 (**A** and **B**) Although pigmentation is common following the treatment of large vessels, these two photos reveal complete destruction of a vessel in the 3 mm in diameter range without pigmentation. Variability such as this makes it difficult to determine the true impact of any treatment strategy

range of sclerosant concentrations (Figs 5.11, 5.12). Compression dressing and hosiery are used to control thrombus size and hopefully reduce hyperpigmentation. Patients with vessels larger than 0.6 mm in diameter can be expected to respond quickly and accordingly can be treated more often, at 1–2-week intervals.

Measuring Veins: The Mechanics

Perhaps the handiest tool of the phlebologist is the No. 30 needle, which at 0.3 mm in diameter is exactly the size above which resistance rarely occurs when treating telangiectasias, and below which resistance is relatively common. The No. 25 needle, at 0.5 mm in diameter, is the size of the vessels that are the bridge between very small vessels, which fade slowly following treatment, and larger vessels that are destroyed suddenly with pigmentation.

Pitfalls in measuring vessels

Stretching the skin

All measurements are best carried out using minimum tension to avoid effacement of very small vessels or increases in vessel diameter produced by tension. For very small vessels, the vessel may be effaced

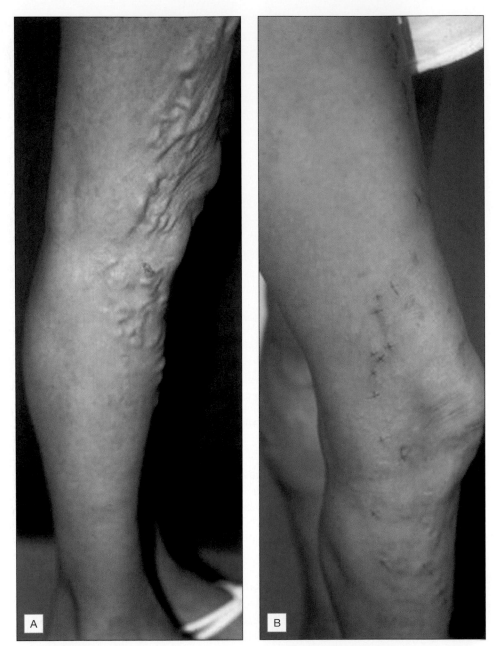

Fig. 5.12 **(A)** This pretreatment photograph demonstrates varicose veins 4–5 mm in diameter. **(B)** 1 week after treatment, almost complete resolution of these veins has occurred associated with minimal pigmentation. These results are a function of intrinsic variability and not particular strategies

by stretching, which makes all vessels somewhat wider. Therefore, measurements may be best made under minimum tension. A generous dab of alcohol renders the skin more transparent, permitting better vessel visibility. A number of devices have been devised that use light to transilluminate deeper vessels, but these are generally not necessary.

Measuring Devices

Biersdorf-Jobst Inc. Charlotte, NC (Tel: 1-800-537-1063) has fabricated an extremely useful clear plastic ruler, which is available directly from the company (Fig. 5.13).

For measuring very small vessels precisely, some form of magnification will be needed, which is also useful when cannulating vessels, which are sometimes smaller than the needle employed. The author prefers Optic-Aids, Mattingly International Inc. (Tel: 1-800-826-4200) (available at Sharper Image), (Fig. 5.14) at about 5×, but other alternatives are feasible, depending on operator preference. Loupes, some with polarizers, and a variety of expensive and more cumbersome devices are also available.

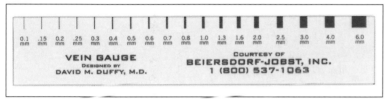

Fig. 5.13 Careful vein measurements are a very effective way of predicting treatment outcomes. This ruler, kindly provided by Biersdorf-Jobst, is a particularly convenient way to carry out these measurements

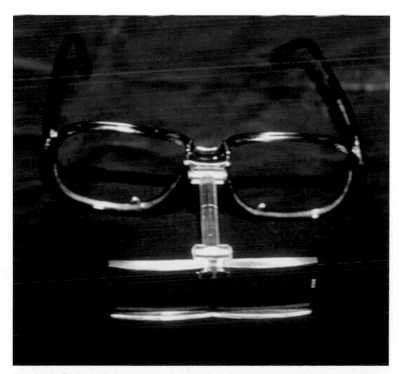

Fig. 5.14 Optic-Aids have proved to be the single most comfortable method of magnifying small vessels

Sclerosants

Sclerosants vary in their profile of advantages and drawbacks. There is no perfect sclerosant (Table 5.1). Sodium sotradecol, polidocanol (aethoxysclerol), and hypertonic saline are the agents most commonly used to treat lower extremity veins. Chromated glycerin, although uncomfortable to use, has also proved quite effective for telangiectasia, and will not produce ulcers on contact (unpublished personal data).

Sclerosants vary in their profile of good and bad characteristics. Hypertonic saline has the advantage of zero occurrence of allergies, however it is extremely technique sensitive; extravasation can produce tissue necrosis in small volumes and at low concentrations. It is also the most uncomfortable to use of all the available sclerosants. Slow injections, followed by a massage, can minimize this discomfort. Polidocanol rarely produces allergies, is painless and appears to be the least toxic or prone to direct contact ulceration of all the detergent sclerosants. Four-tenths of a cc of 3% polidocanol injected into the author's own arm did not produce tissue necrosis (Fig. 5.15). However all sclerosants can produce ulcerations under certain circumstances as revealed in Figure 5.16. Sotradecol, which may be more allergenic than polidocanol, did not produce contact ulcerations when injected at 0.5% concentration into a volunteer, but it did produce ulcers at a 1% concentration. Hypertonic saline can produce ulcerations at a 5% concentration. Deep injections of sclerosing agents did not produce ulcerations, mid-dermal injections did (Fig. 5.17).

Although complications such as matting and hyperpigmentation have been attributed to the type of sclerosant employed, the author's experience suggests that sclerosant concentration and individual variability exert the most important effects. Even more importantly, had treated vessels been carefully measured, the number of parameters affecting outcomes understood, and intrinsic patient variability factored in, arguments regarding some of the putative benefits or drawbacks of a specific type of sclerosant would become moot points. Tables 5.1 and 5.2 present a more detailed comparison of sclerosants. Every phlebologist has his or her own favorites. While in general the potency of any sclerosant is related to its concentration, there remains an absolutely stunning degree of patient-to-patient variation in terms of fragility or resistance to sclerosants (Figs 5.8, 5.9).

Sclerosing Agents/Equivalent Concentrations

By comparing different types and concentrations of commonly used sclerosants side by side on the same patient it has been determined that 0.75% polidocanol is the equivalent of 23.4% hypertonic saline or 0.2–0.3% sotradecol. As a general rule, higher concentrations often will not produce more rapid results in treating telangiectasias ≤ 0.3 mm in diameter, but may result in more matting and occasionally small areas of pigmentation at the site of needle entry. More rapid vessel destruction associated with excessive thrombosis and pigmentation may occur when higher concentrations are used to treat vessels > 0.4 mm in diameter. Lower concentrations are often

Comparison of commonly used sclerosants

Sclerosant/country used	Clinical application (concentration)	Dosage	Advantages	Disadvantages	Complications	Toxicity
Hypertonic saline USA	Abortifacient, spider, small varicose veins (10–30%)	Individual. Restrict volume in patients with salt-restricted diets	Absolute absence of allergies	Moderate discomfort during injection; muscle cramps; generally ineffective for large varicose veins	PE, deaths not reported CTN in concentrations >10%	LD50 in mice NA
Sodium tetradecyl sulfate (Sotradechol, Ikins-Sinn Inc.) USA/worldwide	Varicose and spider veins, esophageal varices (0.1–3%)	Maximum single treatment not to exceed 10 ml	FDA approved in 1946 for varicose veins; Useful for large veins in higher concentrations; Good for smaller vessels in lower concentrations	Mild discomfort on injection; No more effective than saline for small vessels	PE, anaphylaxis, DVT, deaths reported with therapeutic volumes and concentrations CTN at 1% and greater	LD50 in mice 90 ± 5 mg/kg
Sodium morrhuate (Scleromate, Palisades Pharmaceuticals, Inc.) USA/worldwide	Varicose and spider veins; Esophageal varices (5%)	Medium veins 50–100 mg (1–2 ml of 5% injection); Large veins 150–250 mg (3–5 ml of injection)	FDA approved in 1930 for varicose veins	Painful on injection	PE, antigenic, death in therapeutic concentrations and volumes CTN full strength	NA
Ethanolamine oleate (Ethamolin, Glaxo Pharm.) USA/worldwide	Esophageal varices (5%)	Maximum dose: 20 mL of 5%	FDA approved for esophageal varices only in 1989	Allergy	PE, dysphagia, retrosternal pain, esophageal ulcers and strictures, fever, pneumonia, acute renal failure, anaphylaxis, fatal aspiration pneumonia	Minimum lethal intravenous injection in rabbits 130 mg/kg

DVT = deep venous thrombosis, PE = pulmonary embolus, CTN = contact tissue necrosis, NCTN = noncontact tissue necrosis, NA = not available.
Reprinted from Duffy DM Cutaneous necrosis following sclerotherapy. Journal of Aesthetic Dermatology and Cosmetic Surgery 1:157–168

Continued

Table 5.1 Comparison of commonly used sclerosants

Comparison of commonly used sclerosants

Sclerosant/country used	Clinical application (concentration)	Dosage	Advantages	Disadvantages	Complications	Toxicity
Hydroxypolyaethoxydodecan polidocanol (Aethoxysklerol, Globopharm AG) USA/worldwide	Varicose and spider veins, esophageal varices, gastric varices, hemorrhoids (0.5–5%)	Not to exceed 2 mg/kg	Virtually painless to inject; Can be injected into skin without ulcerations; No deaths reported in therapeutic doses or concentrations; Low risk of allergies; No CTN at 3% intradermally*	Transient urticaria and pruritus. Not FDA approved	PE, anaphylaxis, death after overdose (600 mg) caused by pulmonary failure NCTN	
Polyiodide iodine (Variglobin: Sclerodine, Chemische Fabrik, Kreussler Co.,, Germany) Europe /Canada	Varicose veins (2–12%)	Maximum at single session is 3 ml of 6% solution	Allergies not reported	Not FDA approved; Iodine may cause anaphylaxis	PE, CTN reported with paravenous injections; Cutaneous allergies, varicophlebitis	NA
Chromiated glycerin (Scleremo) France	Varicose and spider veins (1.11% chromiated glycerine)	Maximum at single session is 10 ml of pure solution	Low incidence of side effects; No CTN full strength	Not FDA approved; Painful to inject	Necrosis and allergic reaction are very rare; Hematuria	NA

Table 5.1 Comparison of commonly used sclerosants—cont'd

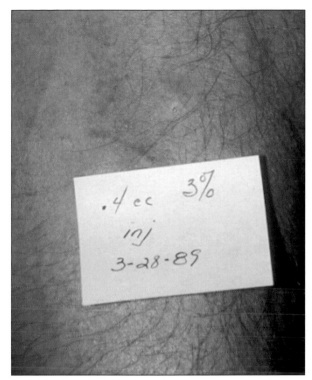

Fig. 5.15 Authors right arm. Direct injection of 3% polidocanol into the mid-dermis did not produce ulceration

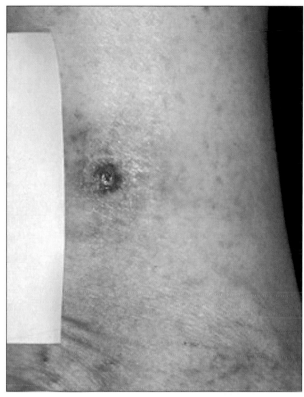

Fig. 5.16 Agents that will not produce tissue necrosis on contact can nevertheless produce ulcers under certain circumstances. In this case in the injection of 0.25% polidocanol was followed by a small ulcer. The ankles are particularly prone to ulceration and these photographs, side-by-side, document the fact that any sclerosant can cause tissue necrosis.

associated with a higher incidence of treatment failures, although as noted earlier certain individuals will develop identical outcomes using both low and high concentrations of sclerosants (Figs 5.7–5.9). Box 5.1 summarizes factors that influence the choice of higher or lower sclerosant concentrations.

FDA Approval

Only sodium sotradecol and sodium morrhuate are FDA approved for the treatment of lower extremity veins. The former was approved in 1946, the latter in the 1920s. Sodium morrhuate may be associated with an unacceptable risk of allergies and tissue necrosis, and is best avoided. Hypertonic saline, approved as an abortifactant can be legally employed as an off-label agent. The decision to use a particular type of sclerosant must take into account both patients' safety and medico-legal liability. Certain insurance carriers will not cover the use of nonFDA-approved medications and in at least one case a physician's license was revoked when he treated patients whose medical insurance specifically prohibited the use of nonFDA-approved agents (personal communication).

Factors affecting choice of sclerosant concentration

Higher concentrations
- Younger patients
- Thick-walled vessels (use palpation)
- Hand/feet/pretibial veins
- Breast veins
- Vessels > 4 mm in diameter to compensate for dilution

Lower concentrations
- Age > 60 years
- 0.6–0.9 mm in diameter elevated spider veins
- Thin-walled vessels
- Easy bruisability
- History of spontaneous bleeding following minor trauma

Box 5.1 Factors affecting choice of sclerosant concentration

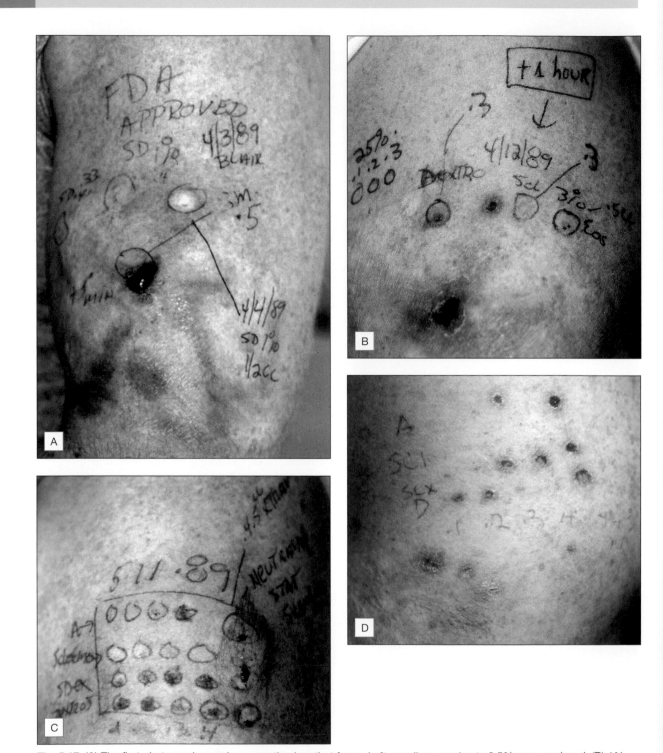

Fig. 5.17 (**A**) The first photograph reveals a necrotic ulcer that formed after sodium morrhuate 0.5% was employed. (**B**) 1% sotradecol (blanched area) produced an ulcer on contact; 0.5% did not. (**C**) Direct testing of the ulcerogenic potential of sclerosants was first carried out in 1989. These injections were placed intradermally and subdermally using multiple sclerosant types, concentrations, and volumes. Neutralization using normal saline was only partially effective. (**D**) Note increasing ulceration with increasing volumes of sclerosants. Subcutaneous injections did not produce ulcers

Parameters at a glance

Size (diameter)	Color	Previous treatments	Surface area	No. TX	Short term results	Pigment and thrombi	Compression reticular veins	TX frequency	Outcome	Sclerosant concentration
0.1–2 mm	Red	No	Small	2–4	Gradual fade	No	Compression sometimes useful	Q 4–6 weeks	Predictable	P = 0.75% HS = 23.4% S = 0.2–0.3%
0.1–0.2 mm	Red	Yes	Large or small	2–6	Gradual fade; resistance common	No	Compression sometimes useful	Q 3–6 months	Variable	P = 0.75% HS = 23.4% S = 0.2–0.3%
0.3 mm	Red	NE	Large or small	2–6	Gradual fade; resistance rare	Rare	Compression sometimes useful	Q 4–6 weeks	Predictable	P = 0.75% HS = 23.4% S = 0.2–0.3%
0.5 mm	Red/magenta	NE	Large or small	1–4[a]	Quick results; resistance rare	50%	Compression & reticular veins sometimes useful	Q 1–2 weeks	Predictable	P = 0.5–0.75% HS = 12.5–23.4% S = 0.2%
0.6–0.9 mm[b]	Magenta/blue–green	NE	Large or small	1–2	Quick results; resistance rare	> 50%	Compression & reticular veins useful	Q 1–2 weeks	Predictable	P = 0.5–0.75% HS = 12.5% S = 0.2%
1–1.6 mm[b]	Blue–green	NE	Large or small	1–2	Quick results; resistance rare	> 50%	Compression useful	Q 1–2 weeks	Predictable	P = 0.75–1.5% HS = 23.4% S = 0.3–0.5%
1.6–2.5 mm[b]	Blue–green	NE	Large or small	1–2	Quick results; resistance rare	> 50%	Compression useful	Q 1–2 weeks	Predictable	P = 1–3% HS = 23.4% S = 0.5–2%
2.5+ mm[b]	Blue–green	NE	Large or small	1–2	Quick results; resistance rare	> 50%	Compression mandatory	Q 1–2 weeks	Predictable	P = 1.5–3% HS = 23.4% S = 0.5–1.5%

NE = No effect, P = Polidocanol, HS = Hypertonic Saline, S = Sotradechol. [a]When vessels 0.1–0.5 mm in diameter occur in large numbers, more treatments may be necessary and the incidence of matting may be increased. [b]Vessels 0.6–0.9 mm in diameter occur commonly in older patients (over 60 years) and may require lower sclerosant concentrations, particularly when vessels are thin walled, elevated or tortuous. When they occur in large numbers, venous reflux may be present. Important notes:. (1) Vessels change color where they cross fascial gaps; (2) Compression and/or reticular vein injections may both decrease number of injection sites and/or minimize thrombi and pigmentation in more fragile vessels; (3) Thin-walled 2.5 mm in diameter vessels involving the lateral thighs/popliteal fossae or located over perforating veins are often a sign of venous reflux, particularly when associated with clusters of elevated tortuous 0.1–1 mm in diameter telangiectasias (corona phlebectasia).

Table 5.2 Parameters at a glance

Compression

Compression dressings and hosiery have been advocated for vessels of all sizes to reduce pigmentation and thrombosis, speed up the treatment process, and produce longer lasting results. Unfortunately compression methods of all types have their own set of problems. Tape dressings occasionally produce allergies and require a waterproof covering when the patient bathes.

All forms of compression are hot and sometimes uncomfortable. In the case of hosiery many problems will occur when it is used to treat patients who have podiatric disorders such as bunions and diabetics with neuropathy. Particular caution is imperative when prescribing compression hosiery for these individuals. Compliance is also a problem. Very few patients will wear this hosiery during the summer months. Pantyhose are associated with vaginal candidiasis, a difficult problem particularly for those who have had previous infections. Some patients complain about abdominal pressure and difficulty breathing. The prescription of thigh-high hosiery, even though it requires garters or It Stays adhesive, AllegroMedical.com, sometimes circumvents both problems. For patients unable to tolerate heavier compression around the feet, it is sometimes beneficial to cut the feet out of the hosiery and stitch the fabric so it does not unravel. This method can only be used when veins are located where compression remains adequate with the hosiery feet removed.

When treating vessels < 2 mm in diameter, the author carried out side-by-side comparisons using compression hosiery on one leg and none on the other. This study involving 50 patients was not able to demonstrate a significant difference in treatment outcomes. As an aside, compression appears to be most useful in treating varicose veins that occur below the knees. Knee-high hosiery, although easy to don and less uncomfortable in hot weather, must be properly fitted to avoid circulatory compromise. When prescribing knee-high hosiery, the physician should ensure the availability of a good fitter and discuss with patients the signs and symptoms of circulatory compromise (numbness, tingling or swelling). When this occurs patients are told to discontinue wearing the hosiery and call the office for advice.

Compression (20–30 mmHg) is routinely used for vessels > 2 mm in diameter, and for patients who are symptomatic, or have obvious reflux. For patients with very fragile vessels (0.6–0.9 mm in diameter), there may be some value in using compression as well. Light compression hosiery (8–20 mmHg) is an excellent adjunct for reducing fatigue and enhancing long-term treatment results for patients whose work requires long periods of standing or sitting. Patients who travel within 2 weeks after treatment are advised to wear hosiery during the travel process, avoid alcohol and drink copious amounts of liquids. When large vessels are treated, patients should be encouraged to take aspirin on these trips. Lawsuits have been filed when patients developed thrombophlebitis or pulmonary emboli on long flights 1–2 weeks after treatment (personal communication).

Clinical Presentations/Outcomes

Patients who present with extensive telangiectasias will often require more treatments, even though every vessel is sclerosed at each treatment session. These patients probably have a defect in the control of vessel growth. Patients with numerous telangiectasias > 0.6 mm in diameter are more likely to have reflux or venous hypertension. Patients who present with small numbers of previously untreated telangiectasias generally enjoy more rapid results, commonly require fewer treatments, and develop less matting or second-generation vessels than those who present with large numbers of telangiectasias.

Common Complications

Hemosiderotic hyperpigmentation

Pigmentation has been attributed to a large number of factors including specific sclerosant types, excessive concentrations, failure to use compression, and skin color. In addition, persistent pigmentation has been ascribed to failure to drain thrombi. The author's experience suggests that pigmentation is:

- Related to vessel size, vessel fragility and rapidity of destruction
- Unavoidable in many patients and is not related to the type of sclerosant employed
- Related to concentration, with higher concentrations sometimes but not always producing increased pigmentation in vessels larger than 0.4 mm in diameter, but only rarely in vessels $\leq$ 0.3 mm in diameter.

Pigmentation of identical severity can occur following the use of sclerosants that vary in concentration by a factor of ten (e.g. 0.125–1.25% polidocanol). Under certain circumstances, narrow linear streaks of pigmentation which follow treatment of small vessels and lie parallel to each other will spread out and coalesce, producing a rectangular macule. A variety of theories have been proposed regarding the etiology of pigmentation that unfortunately fail to explain the fact that pigmentation has never been reported following treatment of veins in certain anatomical sites, ie, hand veins. Temporary hemosiderotic hyperpigmentation, in association with thrombi, frequently occurs, usually resolving between 6 months and 2 years. Q-switched lasers (532–1064 nm) as well as pulsed-dye lasers have been successfully used to treat persistent pigmentation, but generally this is an unnecessary and expensive alternative.

Post-Sclerotherapy Thrombosis/Treatment

The occurrence of palpable, sometimes uncomfortable thrombi is a common event and can lead to a great deal of patient concern and dissatisfaction, including thoughts of: 'Will these break loose?'

Although spontaneous resolution can occur over long periods of time (several months), thrombectomy (incision and drainage) is often employed under local anesthetic using a No. 11 scalpel blade when thrombi are painful or unsightly. Thrombectomy is more easily carried out before thrombi become fibrotic. In most patients this procedure is best performed within 2 weeks after treatment. Although thrombi usually occur quickly after treatment in some individuals, thrombosis can occur spontaneously some 6 weeks post treatment. This phenomenon has important implications in regard to the occurrence of emboli and duration of time necessary for compression. When treating large varicose veins, long distance travel is discouraged for at least 1 month post treatment. Thrombosis and pigmentation are intimately associated with vascular fragility and rapid destruction of vessels. Thrombi can spontaneously resolve without releasing hemolyzed blood into the surrounding tissues (pigmentation) but pigmentation can also occur in the absence of any palpable or visible thrombi. To determine the efficacy of draining thrombi to reduce pigmentation, the author deliberately incised and drained only one-half of the thrombosed veins, leaving the other half intact (Fig. 5.18). In most of the patients treated

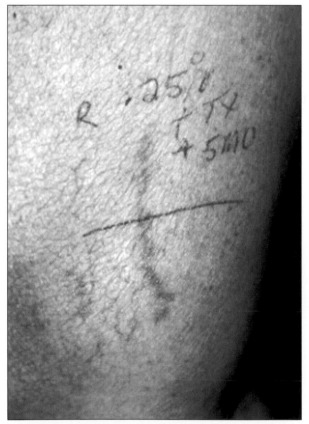

Fig. 5.18 Evacuation of thrombi has been advocated as a means of reducing pigmentation. This photograph reveals the ineffectiveness of draining thrombi in preventing pigmentation. The section of vein below the line was not incised and drained, the upper section was

this way there was no difference in the degree of pigmentation between the incised and unincised areas. Indeed, in some cases intact thrombi resolved without pigmentation. Indeed in 25% of the patients thrombi which had not been treated resolved without pigmentation, whereas the areas that were treated developed more pigmentation.

Long-Term Observations/Proliferation and Involution

In contradistinction to varicose veins, true occurrence of adequately treated telangiectasias is rare. Typically telangiectasias clear after several treatments, when the patient returns several years later a new crop of vessels is noted in roughly the same area. These vessels are often smaller in size and much more resistant to treatment. This is particularly true for telangiectasias involving the inner and outer thighs. Subsequent rounds of treatment will often initiate cycles of involution followed by proliferation of new vessels over many years. The author provides patients with an article that discusses this phenomenon reinforced with clinical photographs.

Matting/Neovascularization/Second-generation Veins

The term 'matting' appeared in 1988, describing very small vessels that occurred after sclerotherapy. In fact, the appearance of small resistant vessels that occur very quickly or long after sclerotherapy may be part of a process of traumatically induced vascular remodeling. Although they look no different and they are often located close to previously treated vessels, they are in fact qualitatively different from the small vessels that in previously untreated patients uniformly responded to treatment (Fig. 5.10).

Matting/Angiogenesis vs. Apoptosis: The Angiogenic Tightrope

No one really knows what causes telangiectasias. Do they represent a defect in inhibitory cytokines, an imbalance in proliferative cytokines, failure of apoptotic processes, or a biomechanical response to abnormal venous hemodynamics? In any event, patients who present with large numbers of spider veins obviously have a problem with control of vessel growth, which is usually tightly regulated. Every time a patient is injected (traumatized), a cumulative effect in promoting angiogenesis may occur. Patients are told that in receiving treatment for small vessels they are walking an angiogenic 'tightrope' in which trauma to targeted vessels and surrounding tissue can produce a rebound in vessel growth. In addition the author discusses the fact that an ideal window of opportunity for good results exists when the patient comes in for the first few rounds of telangiectasia treatment. Patients who seek treatment for very small vessels that remain or have emerged after multiple previous treatments are often disappointed no matter what technique is employed.

The author carried out duplex studies to determine the role of venous reflux in neovascularization. These studies revealed that venous reflux is present in only a small percentage of the patients with significant matting. When reflux was discovered patients who underwent surgery to relieve venous hypertension, sometimes noted an improvement in matting at other times they did not. Since matting can subside spontaneously, there is no way of determining whether patients benefited from surgery or not.

Venous Reflux

Venous reflux and hypertension can produce telangiectasias, as in corona phlebectasia, a process that may involve stimulation of endovenous shear receptors. If the patient prefers, telangiectasia in direct communication with incompetent larger veins may be sclerosed independently with good results. Telangiectasias can also occur in the absence of reflux. Reflux is associated with vessel size and as a general rule many vessels located on the lower extremities that are > 2.5 mm in diameter will exhibit venous reflux on Doppler examination.

Fascial gaps

Fascial gaps consist of palpable depressions beneath reticular veins and telangiectasias where fascia is absent. These gaps permit light transmittal through these vessels and dampening of the Tyndall effect. Gaps are often seen on the lateral thigh and lateral gastrocnemius muscle. Larger reticular veins that cross fascial gaps are sometimes fragile and more prone to pigmentation, and may respond to lower concentrations of sclerosants.

Ulcers

The etiology of sclerotherapy-induced tissue necrosis (ulcers) is poorly understood. All sclerosants are capable of producing tissue necrosis, a phenomenon that can occur following the use of agents that will not produce necrosis on direct contact. Ulcers most commonly occur as a consequence of poor technique and the use of higher sclerosant concentrations. They can occur following extravasation and can also occur despite flawless technique. Premonitory signs consist of persistent blanching (Fig. 5.19) associated in the case of hypertonic saline with a great deal of pain. Another type of ulcer that can be predicted at the time of treatment is unrelated to technique or sclerosant type and may represent injection into an AV malformation or a neurologically mediated vasospastic phenomenon.

Useful ploys in predicting and dealing with tissue necrosis are recognition of precursor signs (petechia and prolonged blanching, or occasionally the occurrence of a very dark ecchymosis). A number of treatments have been advocated. They include flooding the area with normal saline (Fig. 5.20) using 10× the volume assumed to be extravasated. Some authorities advise the injection of hyaluronidase (Wydase). Simple massage or massage using nitroglycerin paste may be effective. Ulcers are much more common on faces and the retromalleolar area (Figs 5.19, 5.16). Low injection force and use of low concentrations are another way to minimize ulceration. Delayed

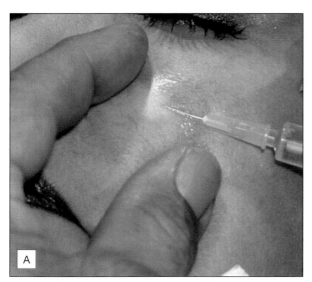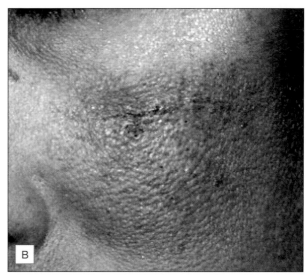

Fig. 5.19 (A) This picture taken during the era when gloves were not employed reveals prolonged blanching following the injection of facial veins, an important sign of an impending ulcer. (B) Ulceration of this kind is another good reason to employ lasers on facial veins, although injections can produce excellent results

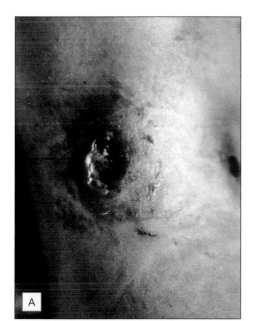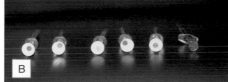

Fig. 5.20 (A) This deep ulceration occurred following the 'neutralization' of extravasated hypertonic saline with more hypertonic saline. (B) Horrific mistakes such as this can be prevented by color coding sclerosant concentrations with these gummed stickers

ulcers can occur without any premonitory signs. Occasionally a patient whose treatment was uneventful will return, describing the development of a scab 4–5 days post treatment, which invariably culminates in the development of an adherent eschar followed by tissue necrosis. Patients are told to inform the treating practitioner if they develop a crust or discomfort any time after the treatment process. When ulcers occur, they can be treated with 5% benzoyl peroxide and DuoDERM or Second Skin. Surgical excision of necrotic ulcers often produces more damage and should be avoided. Careful informed consent and knowledge of the circumstances under which ulcers occur are important both for practitioners and patients.

Questions and Answers

Q: Can telangiectasias be treated any more quickly, efficaciously or with reduction in pigmentation or matting by injecting reticular veins first?

A: This is controversial; I have not found this to be the case in general, although large refluxing reticular veins on the lateral thighs can serve as an excellent conduit enabling the phlebologist to treat large numbers of spider veins simultaneously with fewer injections. In some cases when poor reticular vein–telangiectasia communication is observed, reticular veins can be destroyed, leaving pigment and thrombi without affecting telangiectasias.

Q: Can pigmentation be reduced by compression?

A: Certain patients will or won't develop pigmentation no matter what strategies are employed (Figs 5.11, 5.12, 5.21).

Q: Is postsclerotherapy pigmentation comprised of melanin or hemosiderin?

A: Biopsies have shown that only hemosiderin is present, even in African-American patients. There may be patients in whom postinflammatory pigmentation plays a role.

Q: Will draining thrombi reduce pigmentation?

A: Sometimes it does and in other cases it makes it worse. In many cases it has no effect at all. Thrombi can remain intact for many months and then resorb without pigmentation.

Q: Can telangiectasias be treated more quickly using higher concentrations of sclerosants?

A: Results may be faster for vessels > 0.4 mm in diameter; however, more thrombosis, pigmentation, and matting are commonplace (Figs 5.8, 5.9).

Q: How does the size of the telangiectasia relate to the duration of their presence?

A: Telangiectasias often evolve from very small and red in color, becoming darker (magenta or blue/green) over many years. Elevation and tortuosity also occur during this time frame, and sometimes but not always are associated with venous hypertension. Vessels between 0.6–0.9 mm in diameter (sometimes larger), which are tortuous and elevated above the skin often respond to very low concentrations of sclerosants, and are most commonly

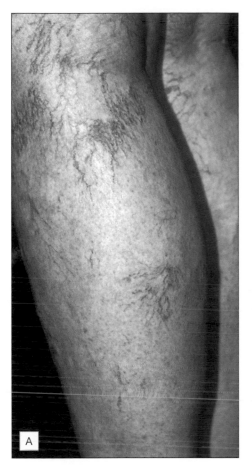 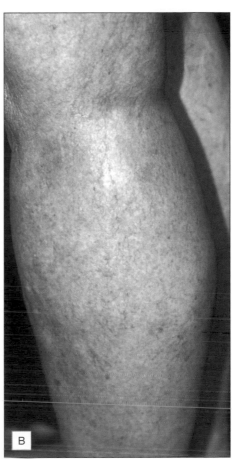

Fig. 5.21 (A) Pretreatment photograph. **(B)** 17 months after treatment these slides reveal an absolute lack of pigmentation in vessels of this size ordinarily associated with this complication. This is another striking example of patient variability

seen in patients over 60 years of age. Perhaps the best example of this phenomenon is corona phlebectasia.

Q: When do you employ compression hosiery and/or dressings, and what do you use?

A: For large vessels I employ Microfoam (3M) tape (in nontape-allergic patients) and Kotex (Kimberly-Clark, Inc.) pads secured with Micropore (3M) tape. I use them for around 1 week. These are followed by day and night compression hosiery for another week or longer. I suspect that once the thrombus is well established and a very firm cord is felt, hosiery is no longer necessary. The author uses 20–30 mmHg compression during the day and TED hosiery at night. Compression is most valuable in symptomatic patients, patients with vessels > 2 mm in diameter, and for vessels located below the knees.

Q: How do you spot-compress tape-allergic patients?

A: Ace bandages are applied over Kotex pads.

Q: What variables other than vessel size impact treatment outcome?

A: Patient age, surface area of involvement, a history of previous treatments, a positive family history of varicose veins, medications such as anticoagulants, recreational and occupational habits (prolonged standing or sitting), exercise patterns and trauma. In addition to the variables mentioned earlier are the presence of venous reflux, use of compression, female hormones, obesity, sclerosant concentration, injection force, anatomical location, vessel wall thickness, depth, and sclerosant volume. Factors associated with extreme vessel fragility include: elevation and tortuosity of small vessels, and intrinsic, unpredictable patterns of patient variability.

Q: Why are there so many disagreements about the ideal way to treat lower extremity veins?

A: Far from being passive conduits for blood flow, human veins and arteries constitute an extraordinarily complex organ system that is involved in the wide variety of physiologic and pathologic processes as diverse as placenta formation, tumor growth, arteriosclerosis, and rheumatoid arthritis. Sclerotherapy and other ablative techniques walk a tightrope between destroying targeted vessels and activating 50 growth modulators (growth factors and inhibitors), which may orchestrate vessel repair or proliferation, defeat attempts to eradicate veins, and confound the clinician.

Q: Are lasers as effective for lower extremity spider veins and small varicose veins?

A: Sclerotherapy is the treatment of choice 90% of the time. Lasers should be used as a backup 10% of the time (Fig. 5.4).

Q: Why do certain physicians advocate the use of lasers for spider veins?

A: This is a complicated issue: (1) Certain types of very small vessels are quite resistant to sclerotherapy, or for that matter any other type of therapy. This resistance is often temporary and when laser treatment occasionally appears to be effective it is hailed as a therapeutic advance in the treatment of these vessels. In fact, by waiting a substantial period of time and then employing sclerotherapy, reasonable results can be achieved. (2) The 'doctor in the toy shop' phenomenon. Doctors like to experiment with new equipment, including lasers, which have a great deal of public cachet. Many manufacturer-funded investigations are still being carried out and in some cases reports dealing with their efficacy are overly optimistic. There is a dearth of careful comparative studies between lasers and sclerotherapy that attribute an advantage to lasers; and (3) The public is fascinated with lasers and demands these supposedly more advanced treatments.

Overall, most laser experts agree that sclerotherapy remains the first-line treatment for treatment of leg veins. Using lasers only when they are appropriate will reduce patient disappointment with treatment.

Q: How do endovenous laser and radiofrequency treatments compare with surgery and sclerotherapy for treatment of large refluxing veins?

A: These modalities appear to offer measurable advantages in certain carefully selected patients over other treatment modalities.

Q: Which new therapies have the potential to treat telangiectasias?

A: Agents that affect the balance between proliferative cytokines and apoptotic processes have been used successfully to treat unwanted vasculature. Imiquimod (Aldara) may have efficacy for treating hemangiomas, possibly by changing cytokine profiles or inducing apoptosis. Anti-vascular endothelial growth factor (VEGF) agents have proved effective for treatment of ocular neovascularization. Imiquimod is sufficiently safe to justify a trial on resistant telangiectasias.

Q: What role do female hormones have in determining responses to sclerotherapy?

A: Female hormones maintain the integrity of vascular endothelium and probably play an important but poorly defined role in a variety of responses to trauma and in the generation of new vessels during periods of hormonal excess.

Treatment Pearls

For small vessels ($\leq$ 0.3 mm in diameter), large (4-fold) increases in sclerosant concentration rarely will speed up resolution, but may increase the incidence of pigmentation and will definitely increase the incidence of neovascularization and ulcers.

Vessels ranging in diameter from 0.5–0.9 mm are sometimes but not always more sensitive to 2-fold increases in sclerosant concentration. For vessels in this size range, a doubling of concentration may result in more rapid destruction and increases in pigment and clotting. For vessels 2 mm in diameter and greater, increases in sclerosant concentration are often necessary to overcome the dilutional effects of high volume blood flow. There are however, patients who have extraordinarily fragile larger vessels. Selection of sclerosant concentration must be done on an individual basis.

Injection Force

Forceful injections, particularly when combined with high concentrations of sclerosants, are a formula for tissue trauma, which will result in increasing neovascularization, pigmentation and ulceration, and will not necessarily speed up the treatment process. When petechiae or severe erythema are noted during the injection process, consider using less injection force and/or lower concentrations of sclerosants.

Selection of Sclerosant Concentration

As a general rule, lower concentrations of sclerosants produce slower results, more treatment failures, and less pigment, thrombosis, inflammation, and matting. For vessels between 0.1 mm and 0.5 mm in diameter, I routinely employ 0.75% polidocanol. For vessels between the diameters of 0.6 mm and 0.9 mm, the concentration may be reduced to 0.5%, particularly in elderly patients where these vessels are elevated or tortuous. A great deal of variability in terms of response to sclerosants can also exist in vessels > 1 mm in diameter. Wall thickness (estimated by palpating the veins), depth, patient age, and location also play a role. Common concentrations are listed in 'Parameters at a glance' (Table 5.2).

Some additional thoughts include the following:

1. Pregnancy has a variable effect upon lower extremity varicose veins and telangiectasias. In general with repeated pregnancies telangiectasias and varicose veins appear earlier and are more severe. This process peaks at the third pregnancy. It is wise to wait at least 6 months postpartum before administering treatment. Veins that appear or worsen during pregnancy may spontaneously resolve.

2. Ask patients to circle the vessels that bother them the most. This approach avoids the phonecall several days later claiming that the vein that the patient wanted treated was 'missed.'

3. Never forget to treat the anterior thighs. Most complaints will come from patients in whom a few small vessels were missed where they are most obvious. Patients often care very little about vessels that involve the posterior leg and thigh.

4. Exercise caution when treating areas in which ulceration has previously occurred. A major danger area is the medial malleolus, and the presence of an adjacent scar caused by a previous ulcer is a further telltale sign.

5. Have an open-door policy for the patient's concerns. Tell patients that they will be seen without charge for a brief examination if they are concerned about the treatment outcome.

6. Warn patients with telangiectasias about increasing resistance with multiple treatments.

7. Do not guarantee results. Talk patients out of compulsively treating every tiny vessel. Explain that more treatments may lead to the appearance of more vessels.

8. Patients with very large vessels and obvious signs of venous insufficiency may not be the best candidates for routine sclerotherapy. When duplex or Doppler ultrasound examinations reveal significant reflux, the author refers these patients to physicians who have their own duplex imaging device and who treat such veins on a daily basis. The younger a symptomatic patient is when she seeks help, the more likely it is that valvular incompetence is to blame. Other signs of valvular insufficiency are corona phlebectasia, a positive family history of varicose veins, or fatigue/aching in association with menstrual cycles.

9. Stress the concept that all patients are different and that each one needs to be treated on an individual basis.

10. Openly discuss the fact that insurance companies should not be asked to compensate patients for cosmetic procedures.

11. Patients will sometimes complain when they think they see more vessels after than before treatment. This is another excellent reason to take photographs to document the pre-treatment appear-

ance. The author explains to these patients that they are finding vessels they never noticed before treatment because they are watching more closely.

12. A primary cause of patient concern is the occurrence of thrombi that they can feel as 'a rock in my sock.' Patients are extremely worried that these clots may break loose. A careful explanation of the lack of danger in these clots coupled with instructions to return for examination when they occur will help allay these concerns.

13. In vessels 0.2 mm in diameter and smaller, check for rapid capillary filling, which when it occurs suggests high flow rates and resistance.

14. A major cause of patient dissatisfaction following sclerotherapy is the occurrence of resistant, small telangiectasias. Typically, patients who experience good results following their first few rounds of treatments attribute bad results following subsequent treatments to poor technique or a different sclerosant. A careful explanation of the difference between virgin (previously untreated) telangiectasia and second-generation vessels will avoid patient dissatisfaction with treatment outcomes. The current author uses different treatment frequencies for previously treated patients with small vessels as noted in 'Parameters at a glance' (Table 5.2).

15. It is generally appropriate to obtain duplex scanning for any patient who is symptomatic, has Doppler evidence of junctional insufficiency, has veins larger than 5 mm in diameter, or has severe corona phlebectasia. Doppler or duplex examinations are not routinely performed on patients who present simply for spider veins and small reticular veins.

16. Sclerotherapy is best suited for the treatment of vessels between 0.3 mm and 5 mm in diameter. Vessels smaller than 0.3 mm in diameter have a high incidence of resistance to treatment. Larger veins can be treated effectively by experienced phlebologists.

17. Tell patients there is no cure for varicose veins or telangiectasias. Repeated treatments may be necessary and wearing support hosiery can help.

18. When the concentration of sclerosant is too low, the result will often be thrombosis of only a short proximal segment of the treated vessel.

19. Give your patients orange juice or fruit if they have not eaten for more than 4 hours to avoid vasovagal reflexes.

20. Paper examination shorts (Distributed by McKesson General Medical Corp. (800) 755-2090), and Edroy OpticAids – 5 diopter (Distributed by Mattingly International, Inc. (800) 826-4200) are very useful and inexpensive.

21. Sanitary napkins make excellent compression dressings when used with tape or hosiery.

22. When patients complain of pruritus immediately after injections (most commonly around the ankles), the application of ice bags (e.g. Instant Cold Compresses, McKesson Medical-Surgical, Richmond, VA) will stop the itching almost immediately.

23. Beware of the patient with a very high pain tolerance, particularly when using hypertonic saline. These patients may ignore what they regard as minor discomfort. They should be told that they should not be feeling much pain during the process. Patients with a high pain tolerance often will not report problems because they fail to notice them.

24. Superficial thrombophlebitis responds very well to intralesional injections of 2.5 mg per cc of triamcinolone acetonide (Kenalog). This can be injected together with local anesthetic at the time thrombi are incised. If thrombophlebitis occurs in the absence of thrombi, simply inject the intralesional steroid into the areas of tenderness. Pseudoatrophy is rare.

25. Photos and patient instructions are wonderful handouts transforming patients into allies with realistic expectations.

26. Consider giving patients detailed instructions for every aspect of sclerotherapy including compression, when and why it is used, as well as photographs that include commonly observed patterns of response and minor complications. The author originally provided patients with rulers so they could self-assess possible treatment outcomes. This ploy was only partly successful because many patients seemed unable to accurately measure their own veins. It has been found more useful to send a pamphlet describing treatment patterns to all new patients along with a detailed history to be filled out at home. Patients who come to the office with this information and the forms filled out can be accommodated more efficiently.

27. Certain anatomical areas are prone to good or bad results. The posterior thigh is a particularly satisfying area to treat vessels of all sizes. Excellent long term results are the rule, resistant telangiectasia are uncommon. The ankles and face are most prone to ulcers. The inner and outer thighs are most prone to matting. Vessels $\geq$ 2 mm in diameter on the shins often require higher concentrations of sclerosants as do veins on the hand. Reticular veins involving the breast typically appear after breast implantation and are easily treated. Facial telangiectasias are often best treated with lasers. Larger (0.6–1.3 mm in diameter) facial veins can be treated with injections but may be more prone to tissue necrosis. Site-specific results may be due to vascular endothelium heterogeneity.

28. Recurrences are very rare. What is usually called a recurrence is actually a new vessel in roughly the same area. Careful photography will make this clear.

29. Publications the author has found useful are available to interested physicians at info@drdavidmduffy. com (Table 5.1)

Conclusion

Success or failure in the treatment of vessels of all sizes has more to do with intrinsic factors than the choice of any combination of specific therapies. Although there is general agreement among experts regarding the guidelines of treatment of varicose veins, very little agreement exists as to the best way to treat telangiectasias. The author's experience suggests that good or bad results can occur using any treatment protocol largely as a result of patient variability.

Acknowledgments

I'd like to acknowledge the help of Peggy Goodwin, and the patience of my staff, which has been invaluable. Dr Mary P. Lupo should also be acknowledged for her keen powers of observation in relating vessel size and color to the occurrence of pigmentation. Finally, the contributions of four people – Mitchell Goldman, Robert and Margaret Weiss and Neil Sadick – cannot be ignored. These four individuals have produced more useful information in the last decade than has been published in the preceding century.

Further reading

Bergan J, Weiss R, Goldman M 2000 Extensive tissue necrosis following high-concentration sclerotherapy for varicose veins. Dermatologic Surgery 26:535–542

Cabrera J, Cabrera J Jr 2000 Treatment of varicose long saphenous veins with sclerosant in microfoam form. Long-term outcomes. Phlebology 15:19–23

Cabrera J, Cabrera J Jr, Garcia-Olmedo MA et al 2003 Treatment of venous malformations with sclerosant in microfoam form. Archives of Dermatology 139:1409–1416

Davis L, Duffy D 1990 Determination of incidence and risk factors for post-sclerotherapy telangiectatic matting of the lower extremity: A retrospective analysis. Journal of Dermatologic Surgery and Oncology 16:327–330

Dover JS, Sadick NS, Goldman MP 1999 The role of lasers and light sources in the treatment of leg veins. Dermatologic Surgery 25:328–336

Duffy D, Garcia C, Clark RE 1999 The role of sclerotherapy in abnormal varicose hand veins. Journal of Plastic and Reconstructive Surgery 104:1474–1479

Duffy D 1988 Small vessel sclerotherapy: An overview. Advances in Dermatology 3:221

Duffy DM 1996 Second-generation telangiectasia often resists repeat Tx. Dermatology Times

Duffy DM 1998 Sclerotherapy induced vascular remodeling/neovascularization. Phlebology Digest October:6–11

Duffy DM 1999 Cutaneous necrosis following sclerotherapy. Journal of Aesthetic Dermatology and Cosmetic Surgery 1:157–168

Duffy DM 1999 Complications of sclerotherapy for vessels involving the hands and face. Aesthetic Dermatology and Cosmetic Surgery 1:91–93

Duffy D 1999 Techniques of small vessel sclerotherapy. In: Goldman M, Weiss R, Bergna J (eds) Varicose veins and telangiectasia: diagnosis and treatment. 2nd edn. Quality Medical Publishing, St Louis, MO pp 518–547

Duffy DM 2000 How to educate patients about sclerotherapy. Skin and Aging October: 30–37

Duffy D 2002 Vessel size: An excellent prognosticator of clinical outcomes following sclerotherapy. Presented at Hugh Greenways' Superficial Anatomy and Cutaneous Surgery. July 15–20, La Jolla, CA

Duffy DM 2004 Lasers and IPL for lower extremity leg veins: Last resort or promising alternative PowerPoint presentation. ASCDAS December 2004, Phoenix, AZ

Duffy DM, Goldman MP, Kaplan RP 1987 Post-sclerotherapy hyperpigmentation. A histologic evaluation. Journal of Dermatologic Surgery and Oncology May; 13(5):547–550

Evan G, Littlewood T 1998 Apoptosis: A matter of life and cell death. Science Magazine 281:1317–1321

Ferris FL 2004 A new treatment for ocular neovascularization. New England Journal of Medicine 351:2863–2865

Folkman J 1995 Clinical applications of research on angiogenesis. Seminars in medicine of the Beth Israel Hospital, Boston, MA. New England Journal of Medicine 333:1757–1763

Gibbons GH, Dzau VT 1994 The emerging concept of vascular remodeling. New England Journal of Medicine 330:1431–1438

Goldman MP, Bergan JJ 2001 Sclerotherapy: Treatment of varicose and telangiectatic leg veins. 3rd Edn. Mosby St Louis, MO

Green D 1998 Reticular veins, incompetent reticular veins and their relationship to telangiectases. Journal of Dermatologic Surgery 24:1129–1141

Hamel-Desnos C, Desnos P, Wollmann JC, et al 2003 Evaluation of the efficacy of polidocanol in form of foam compared to liquid form in sclerotherapy of the greater saphenous vein: initial results. Dermatologic Surgery 29:1170–1175

Katz B 1998 Laser therapy and sclerotherapy in the treatment of laser and small spider veins. Cosmetic Dermatology September:34–41

Puissegur Lupo ML 1989 Sclerotherapy: review of results and complications in 200 patients. Journal of Dermatologic Surgery and Oncology 15:214–219

Richard James Inc. 2 Centennial Dr, Peabody, MA 01960 Tel: (978) 532-0666 MAXFLO NEEDLES 30 gauge

Sadick NS 1999 Estrogen and progesterone receptors: Their role in postsclerotherapy angio-genesis telangiectatic matting. Dermatologic Surgery 25:539–543

Sadick NS 2000 Manual of sclerotherapy. Lippincott Williams & Wilkins, Philadelphia, PA

Thorin E, Shato MA, Shreeve SM, et al 1998 Human vascular endothelium heterogeneity: A comparative study of cerebral and peripheral cultured vascular endothelial cells. The Yearbook of Vascular Surgery: 56

Weiss R, Duffy D 1999 Clinical benefits of lightweight compression: Reduction of venous-related symptoms by ready-to-wear lightweight gradient compression hosiery. Dermatologic Surgery 25:701–704

Weiss R, Weiss M 1997 Combination intense pulsed light and sclerotherapy: A synergistic effect. Dermatologic Surgery 24:969

Weiss RA, Weiss MA 2000 Vein diagnosis and treatment: A comprehensive approach. Nov. McGraw Hill ISBN 0070692017

Weiss R 1998 Easy to use long-pulse Nd:YAG laser targets selected leg veins. Dermatology Times October:48

Welsh O, Olazaran Z, Gomez M, Salas J, Berman B 2004 Treatment of infantile hemangiomas with short-term applications of imiquimod 5% cream. Journal of the American Academy of Dermatologists 51:639–642

Wickelgren I 1989 The mechanics of natural success. Science News 135:376–378

Wollmann J-CGR 2004 The history of sclerosing foams. Dermatologic Surgery 30:694–703

www.sigmadldrich.com. Anti-tumor agents by mechanisms of action. 3/18/04

Zimmet SE 1996 Hyaluronidase in the prevention of sclerotherapy-induced extravasation necrosis: A dose response study. Dermatologic Surgery 22:73

Laser Surgery

6

Melissa A. Bogle, Neil S. Sadick

Introduction

The problem being treated

Prominent leg veins affect as many as 41% of women and 15% of men in the United States. Vascular pathology can be divided into superficial spider veins or telangiectasias, deeper reticular veins, and protuberant varicosities (Fig. 6.1). Causes include heredity, hormones, prolonged

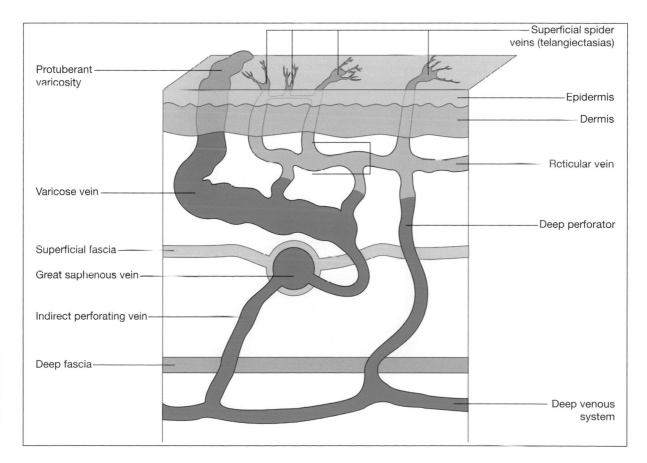

Fig. 6.1 Diagram illustrating types of leg veins including superficial spider veins (telangiectasias), deeper reticular veins, and protuberant varicosities. (Adapted from: Somjen GM et al 1993 Anatomical examination of leg telangiectasias with duplex scanning. Journal of Dermatologic Surgery and Gynecology 19:940)

standing, obesity, pregnancy and aging. Although leg veins may cause symptoms such as fatigue, aching, swelling, throbbing and pain, treatment is sought mainly because of their unsightly appearance.

The venous system of the lower extremity is composed of a complex, interconnected superficial and deep plexus. The superficial veins lie just beneath the skin, and the deep veins travel within the muscles of the leg. Because of flow patterns between the two networks, superficial spider veins may be the result of increased pressure in deeper reticular or varicose veins.

The variety of sizes, depths, flow patterns, and vessel thickness make the treatment of leg veins much more difficult than treatment of facial veins. One important consideration is that even the fine, relatively superficial telangiectatic vessels of the legs are not very close to the surface of the skin, like facial veins, but rather can lie at a depth of up to several millimeters; adverse events and incomplete response may result as laser energy is dissipated in the overlying skin with only partial effect permeating to the targeted vessels (Fig. 6.2). There is no single treatment for all leg veins and lasers may be used as adjunctive therapy in patients receiving sclerotherapy, phlebectomy or vein stripping.

Laser therapy is particularly useful for the treatment of small spider veins or telangiectasias (< 0.5 mm) and in the treatment of telangiectatic matting resulting from other modes of treatment. It can also be used in the treatment of large spider and reticular veins, however sclerotherapy remains the gold standard for treatment of these vessels. Varicose veins are best treated with surgical excision or endovenous ablation (Box 6.1). This chapter will deal only with laser surgery; sclerotherapy, surgical excision, and endovenous ablation are discussed elsewhere in this book.

> ### Treatments of choice for various types of leg veins
>
> - **Small telangiectasias**: laser or sclerotherapy
> - **Telangiectatic matting**: laser or sclerotherapy
> - **Large spider veins, reticular veins**: sclerotherapy
> - **Varicose veins**: surgical excision, endovenous ablation

Box 6.1 Treatments of choice for various types of leg veins

Patient Selection

Laser treatment is most effective for small, superficial red or blue veins. It is an ideal therapy for patients who are prone to telangiectatic matting, do not respond to sclerotherapy, or are fearful of needles.

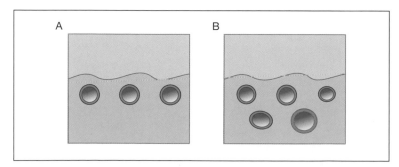

Fig. 6.2 Comparative diagram of differences between facial vessels and telangiectatic leg veins. (**A**) Facial telangiectasias are of a more homogeneous depth than those on the legs, with thinner, more uniform walls and low hydrostatic pressure. (**B**) Leg telangiectasias are deeper with a less uniform depth, thicker walls, and increased hydrostatic pressure

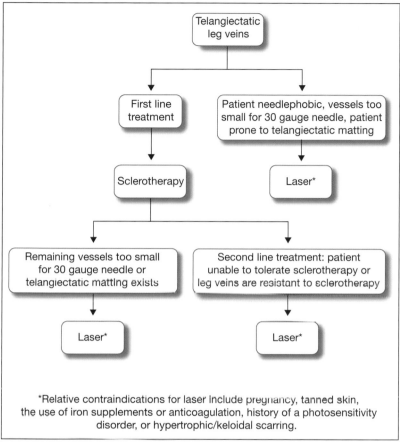

Fig. 6.3 Guidelines for appropriate use of laser vs. sclerotherapy for the treatment of telangiectatic leg veins

Relative contraindications to laser surgery include pregnancy, tanned skin, the use of iron supplements or anticoagulation, history of a photosensitivity disorder, or hypertrophic/keloidal scarring (Fig. 6.3).

Expected Benefits

Laser therapy is an effective modality for the treatment of leg veins. In general, small telangiectatic vessels often disappear at the time of treatment, providing the patient and physician with a visual record of success. Larger telangiectasias and reticular veins typically do not disappear at the time of treatment, but will gradually improve over the course of several months. Selected vessels may clinically darken after treatment as the blood in the vessels coagulates.

In a recent study by Sadick (2003) treating reticular and spider telangiectasias on the lower legs using the monomodal approach with the 1064 nm Nd:Yag laser and variable spot sizes and pulse width parameters, approximately 20% of treated vessels had a 50–75% improvement after three treatments spaced 1 month apart (Fig. 6.4).

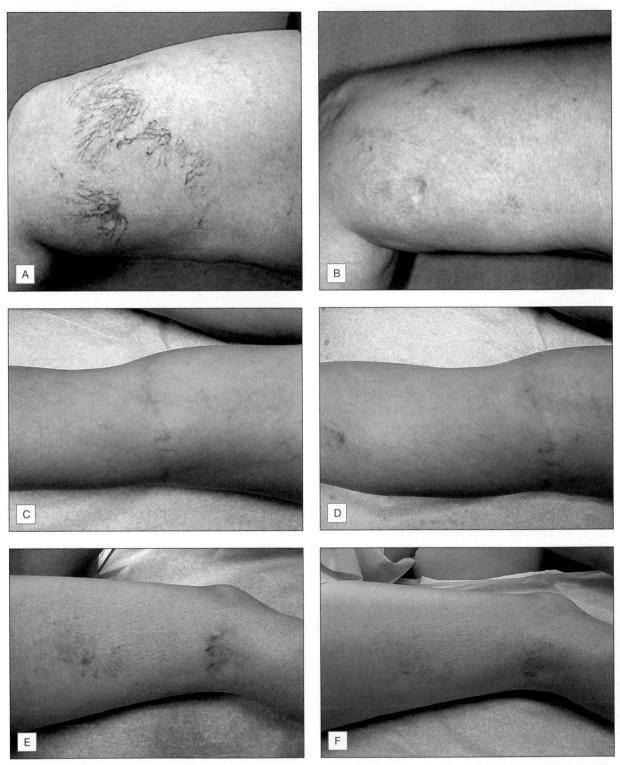

Fig. 6.4 Figures to the right show good resolution of leg veins following three treatments using the 1064 nm Nd:Yag laser with the variate monomodal approach. Figures on the left are pre-treatment. (**A, B**) Patient 1. (**C, D**) Patient 2. (**E, F**) Patient 3

Improvements continued over time, with 80% of vessels having greater than 75% clearing at 6 months follow up. Of the patients treated, 90% were highly satisfied with the treatment.

In a comparative study by Eremia and Umar of the 1064 nm Nd:Yag, 810 nm diode, and 755 nm Alexandrite lasers for the treatment of leg veins measuring 0.3–3 mm in diameter, the Nd:Yag laser was associated with the greatest percent improvement at 3 months' follow up (Table 6.1). Purpura and matting were problematic with the Alexandrite laser, and results with the long-pulsed diode were unpredictable among the 22 women in the study. No long-term controlled studies have been carried out regarding the persistence of vessel clearing after laser treatment of the legs.

Problems intrinsic to the use of lasers for the treatment of leg veins include the need for multiple treatments, patient discomfort, inconsistent results, and high equipment cost. Reported complications include transient hyperpigmentation, purpura, epidermal surface change, telangiectatic matting and thrombus formation. When a systematic approach is used, sclerotherapy can treat 80–90% of vessels in a single treatment. Because of the relatively low cost of venous surgery and sclerotherapy, lasers are generally not recommended as first-line treatment.

Overview of Treatment Strategy

Treatment approach

A detailed physical examination should be performed on all patients presenting for the treatment of leg veins to evaluate the type and size of venous pathology and the presence of reflux or incompetent valves. Large varicose veins showing reflux must be addressed first to avoid unsuccessful treatment of smaller telangiectasias and potential complications such as dyspigmentation and telangiectatic matting.

The treatment of leg veins should follow a systematic approach (Fig. 6.5). First, varicosities and large feeder vessels should be surgically removed (by ligation, stripping, or ambulatory phlebectomy) or treated with endovenous closure. Sclerotherapy should then be performed proceeding from large to small vessels. This will clear on approximately 80–90% of vessels in a single treatment. Laser and light therapy should be used to treat any remaining vessels and those that are too small to reasonably undergo sclerotherapy with a 30–32 gauge needle.

Major determinants

Lasers in the treatment of leg veins follow the principles of selective photothermolysis (Box 6.2). The major parameters that must be chosen to treat an individual vessel include wavelength, pulse duration, and spot size (Table 6.2).

The absorption spectrum of hemoglobin has major peaks at 410, 540, and 577 nm, with smaller peaks at 920–940 nm. Blue veins

Comparison of the 1064 nm Nd:Yag, 810 nm diode, and 755 nm Alexandrite lasers for leg veins measuring 0.3–3 mm in diameter	
Laser	**Patients achieving 75% clearance at 3 months**
1064 nm Nd:Yag	88%
810 nm diode	29%
755 nm Alexandrite	33%

(Reproduced from Eremia S, Li C, Umar SH 2002 A side-by-side comparative study of 1,064 nm Nd:Yag, 810 nm diode and 755 nm alexandrite for treatment of 0.3 3 mm leg veins. Dermatologic Surgery 28:224–230)

Table 6.1 Comparison of the 1064 nm Nd:Yag, 810 nm diode, and 755 nm Alexandrite lasers for leg veins measuring 0.3–3 mm in diameter

Fundamental properties of laser use for leg veins

- The ideal laser must have a wavelength proportionately better absorbed by hemoglobin than the surrounding tissue
- Penetration should reach the full depth of the target vessel
- Sufficient energy must be delivered to damage the vessel without damaging the overlying skin
- Energy must be delivered over an exposure time long enough to slowly coagulate the vessel without damaging surrounding tissue

Box 6.2 Fundamental properties of laser use for leg veins

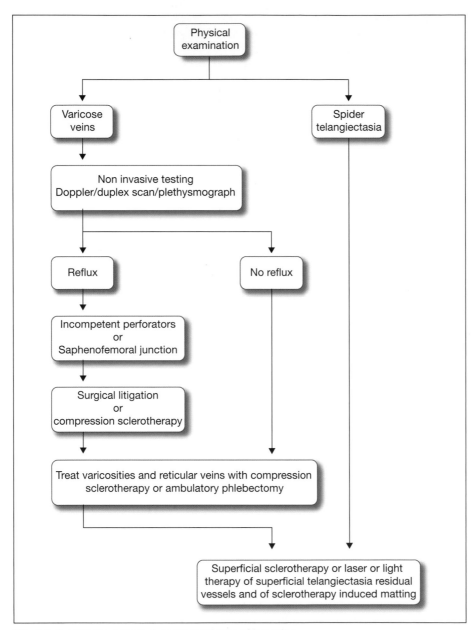

Fig. 6.5 Systematic approach to the treatment of leg veins

Optimal laser parameters for the treatment of leg veins	
Wavelength	530–1064 nm
Pulse duration	2–100 ms
Fluence	30–150 J/cm^2
Spot size	1.5–10 mm

Table 6.2 Optimal laser parameters for the treatment of leg veins

respond better to wavelengths targeting the deoxyhemoglobin spectrum and red veins respond better to wavelengths targeting the oxyhemoglobin spectrum (Fig. 6.6). Absorption by hemoglobin in the long visible to near infrared range is important for vessels > 0.5 mm in diameter and at least 0.5 mm below the skin surface.

Depth of penetration of the laser beam is dependent upon the wavelength and degree of scattering and absorption by the surrounding skin. Longer wavelengths generally have decreased scattering and greater penetration into the skin. Thus, deeper vessels necessitate a longer wavelength to allow penetration to their depth. Likewise, larger spot sizes penetrate deeper into the skin to optimize energy delivery to the vein, and larger vessel diameters require longer pulse durations to slowly and effectively heat the entire vessel.

The earlier mentioned characteristics lead to the development of a bimodal, dual-wavelength approach for the treatment of both red and blue lower extremity veins. Short wavelengths (500–600 nm) were found to be most effective for the treatment of small, reddish telangiectasias with a high degree of oxyhemoglobin. Longer wavelengths (800–1100 nm) were found to be most effective for the treatment of deeper, blue telangiectasias and reticular veins. The downside to this approach is that multiple laser systems must be used to obtain optimal results.

The modified monomodal approach addresses differences in vessel size and depth with a single 1064 nm Nd:Yag laser (Table 6.3). Fine, red vessels < 1 mm in diameter are generally superficial and have a high oxyhemoglobin saturation; they can be effectively treated with small spot sizes (< 2 mm), high fluences (350–600 J/cm^2), and short pulse durations (15–30 ms). Larger blue vessels 1–4 mm in diameter are deeper and have a lower oxygenated hemoglobin component; they can effectively be treated with larger spot sizes (2–8 mm), moderate fluences (100–350 J/cm^2), and longer pulse durations (30–50 ms).

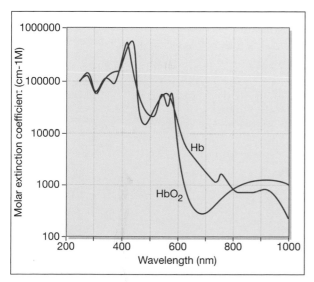

Fig. 6.6 Absorption spectrum of hemoglobin/deoxyhemoglobin

Monomodal approach to the treatment of leg veins using the 1064 nm Nd:Yag laser			
Vessel size	**Spot size**	**Fluence**	**Pulse duration**
< 1 mm (red)	Small	High	Short
1–3 mm (blue)	Large	Moderate	Long

Table 6.3 Monomodal approach to the treatment of leg veins using the 1064 nm Nd:Yag laser

Patient Interviews

Diagnosis of spider or varicose veins begins with a thorough medical history detailing potential risk factors or sources of pathologic leg veins such as heredity, hormones, prolonged standing, obesity, pregnancy, or aging. A detailed physical examination should be carried out while the patient is standing. Pre-existing epidermal pigmentation and the size and type of abnormal veins on both legs should be noted. A hand-held Doppler ultrasound device is used to map the leg veins and determine the direction of blood flow. If there is reflux or backward flow, the patient requires further testing with a duplex ultrasound (DUS) machine. It is important for patients not only to be thoroughly evaluated during their initial visit but also to be clearly instructed regarding the most appropriate treatment approach, whether this requires surgery, sclerotherapy, lasers, or combined treatments.

Treatment Techniques

Patients

Ideal candidates for laser treatment of leg veins have undergone appropriate surgery or sclerotherapy for the treatment of varicosities, incompetent perforators and reticular veins, as well as sclerotherapy to clear the majority of superficial vessels.

Laser therapy of leg veins may be considered prior to sclerotherapy in patients who: (1) are fearful of needles; (2) do not tolerate sclerotherapy; (3) have leg veins unresponsive to sclerotherapy; or (4) are prone to telangiectatic matting (Box 6.3).

Equipment

Numerous lasers are available for treatment of leg veins (Tables 6.4 and 6.5). The first laser to achieve reasonable results in the treatment of leg veins was the pulsed-dye laser in the 1980s. Although the wavelength was able to penetrate deep enough to treat fine, superficial telangiectasias, the pulse duration was too short to effectively damage larger vessels. Side effects included bruising and post-therapy hyperpigmentation.

Ideal patient characteristics
■ Leg veins are resistant to sclerotherapy
■ Patient does not tolerate sclerotherapy
■ Patient is fearful of needles
■ Patient is prone to telangiectatic matting
■ Vessels smaller than the diameter of a 30 gauge needle are present

Box 6.3 Ideal patient characteristics

Lasers and light sources for the treatment of leg veins	
Laser	**Wavelength**
Pulsed dye	585–605 nm
KTP	532 nm
Alexandrite	755 nm
Diode	810 nm
Nd:Yag	1064 nm
Intense pulsed light	515–1200 nm

Table 6.4 Lasers and light sources for the treatment of leg veins

Lasers available for treatment of leg veins

Device	Clinical use	Common settings
Pulsed dye laser	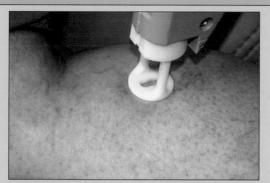	16–20 J/cm², 3×10 mm elliptical spot, 10–20 msec, 50/20 DCD (Vbeam, Candela Corp, Wayland, MA)
KTP laser	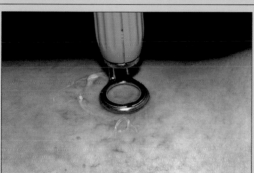	12–20 J/cm², 3–5 mm spot, 10–15 ms, sapphire contact cooling (Gemini, Laserscope, San Jose, CA)
Alexandrite laser	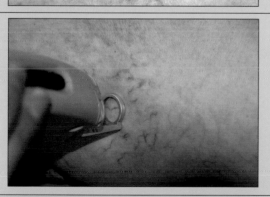	70 J/cm², 8 mm spot, 3 ms, 70/20 DCD (GentleLase, Candela Corp, Wayland, MA)
Nd:YAG laser	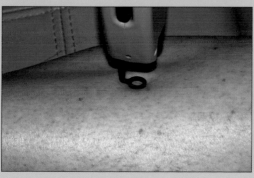	450–500 J/cm²,1.5 mm spot, 60 ms, 50/20/10 DCD *or* 230–300 J/cm², 3 mm spot, 60 ms, 50/20/10 DCD for vessels <1 mm in diameter. Reticular veins should use lower energy, starting at 180 J/cm². Avoid pulsing telangiectasia over reticular veins as depressions and scarring may occur (GentleYAG. Candela Corp, Wayland, MA)

Table 6.5 Lasers available for treatment of leg veins

Continued

Lasers available for treatment of leg veins—cont'd		
Device	**Clinical use**	**Common settings**
Intense pulsed light	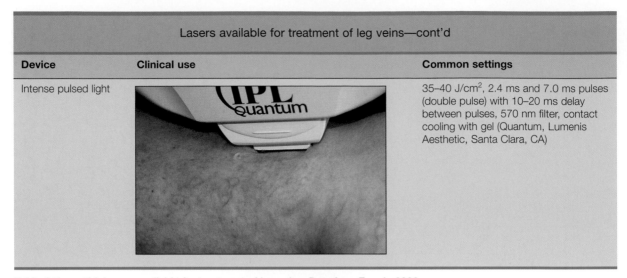	35–40 J/cm², 2.4 ms and 7.0 ms pulses (double pulse) with 10–20 ms delay between pulses, 570 nm filter, contact cooling with gel (Quantum, Lumenis Aesthetic, Santa Clara, CA)

Table 6.5, cont'd Lasers available for treatment of leg veins. Data from Eremia 2002

The recent development of longer wavelength, longer pulse duration lasers and light sources has greatly improved treatment outcomes, and most lasers have incorporated cooling mechanisms to protect the epidermis at higher fluences. Currently several long-pulse dye lasers are available with variable pulse durations capable of deeper penetration into the skin and treatment of larger superficial telangiectasias. The pulse duration most suited for the thermal destruction of leg telangiectasias appears to be 1–50 ms. However, it remains important to counsel patients that purpura lasting several weeks may occur. Hyperpigmentation, if it occurs, may take several months to fade.

KTP lasers are effective for small telangiectatic leg veins in fair-skinned patients. The most positive results have been achieved by using 3–5 mm spot sizes, 10–15 ms pulse durations, and fluences of 14–20 J/cm² (Aura; Laserscope, San Jose, CA). Temporary redness and superficial crusting is common, however purpura is rare. Because melanin also absorbs green light well, darker skinned patients are limited to lower fluences, which may not be enough to successfully coagulate the vessel. As when this laser is used for facial vessels, it is important to avoid multiple passes at relatively high fluences; the lack of marked immediate tissue effect can mask the fact that such repeated pulses may result in epidermal damage that can eventually heal with textural change or indentation of the overlying skin (Fig. 6.7).

Other lasers used for leg veins include the long-pulse Alexandrite, diode lasers and long-pulse Nd:YAG laser. Longer wavelengths, deeper penetration, and fair absorption by hemoglobin make them suitable for large telangiectatic and deep reticular veins. In addition, longer wavelengths have less interaction with epidermal melanin, allowing safer treatment of leg veins in darker skin types. The most favorable treatment parameters for long-pulse Alexandrite lasers appear to be

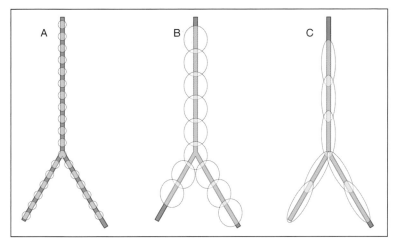

Fig. 6.7 (**A**) The one pass approach with the KTP or 1064 nm lasers involve tracing the vessel with nonoverlapping pulses to avoid excessive thermal damage. (**B**, **C**) The long-pulsed Alexandrite and pulsed-dye lasers may overlap by approximately 15–20% and multiple passes may be performed, if needed

20 J/cm^2, double pulsed at a repetition rate of 1 Hz. Side effects include purpura, matting, and long-term pigmentary alterations due to melanin absorption.

The long-pulse Nd:YAG laser is considered to be the laser of choice for the treatment of leg veins. As discussed earlier in this chapter, spot sizes, energy and pulse duration can be fine-tuned to target both small telangiectasias and larger reticular veins with a single device. In addition, issues stemming from the hydrostatic pressure of feeder and reticular veins can be addressed because veins up to 3 mm in diameter can be treated, although pain becomes an issue with large vessels. For superficial vessels less than 1 mm in diameter, small spot sizes (less than 2 mm), short-pulse durations (15–30 ms), and high fluences (350–600 J/cm^2) are optimal (Lyra; Laserscope, San Jose, CA). For reticular veins 1–4 mm in diameter, larger spot sizes (2–8 mm), longer pulse durations (30–60 ms) and moderate fluences (100–370 J/cm^2) should yield successful results (Lyra; Laserscope, San Jose, CA).

Intense pulsed-light devices have also been reported for the treatment of leg veins, however results have been variable. These devices emit noncoherent light with wavelengths between 500–1200 nm in single, double, or triple pulses. The longer wavelengths can penetrate deep into the skin to coagulate deeper vessels. Commonly, 550 and 570 nm filters are appropriate to deliver primarily yellow and red wavelengths with some infrared component. While the large spot size with this device is advantageous, in some hands, an unacceptable rate of side effects has been reported, including blistering, crusting, and discoloration, especially in darker skinned patients.

A newly developed technology in the treatment of leg veins is the combination of bipolar radiofrequency and optical energy, using either the diode laser or an intense pulsed-light source. It is thought that the two forms of energy may act synergistically to achieve a greater target effect. The laser component selectively heats the vessel, allowing the preferential absorption of radiofrequency energy because of the increased temperature and high electrical conductivity of blood. Preliminary studies by Sadick (2005) using a 915 nm diode laser with radiofrequency energy show 30% of patients achieving greater than 75% vessel clearance and 78% of patients achieving greater than 50% clearance of their leg veins in one to three treatments.

Treatment algorithm

Most patients tolerate laser surgery for leg veins without difficulty. If the patient is sensitive or if larger telangiectasias or reticular veins are to be treated, a topical anesthetic cream should be applied 1 hour before treatment and covered with plastic wrap. In some instances, treatment of reticular veins can be associated with significant discomfort, including a deeper, more intense pain that is below the level of effect of topical anesthetic. As long as patients are advised of this in advance, virtually all are able to complete treatment with additional anesthesia. When the patient and physician are ready to begin, the treatment area should be cleansed with alcohol and the physician, patient and any assistants should don appropriate protective eyewear.

When treating smaller telangiectasias with the 532 nm KTP laser, fluences of 12–20 J/cm^2 delivered with a spot size of 3–5 mm and a pulse duration of 10–15 ms yield the best results (Aura; Laserscope, San Jose, CA). Skin cooling should be used before, during, and after treatment to prevent thermal damage to surrounding tissues and decrease patient discomfort. Individual laser pulses separated by at least 1–2 mm should then be traced along the length of the vein, with the operator being careful not to overlap or double pulse (Fig. 6.7). It is important to apply only minimal pressure with the hand piece so as not to physically compress the target vessel (Fig. 6.8). The treatment goal should be either vessel spasm with immediate clearance or thrombosis with darkening of the vessel. Although complete resolution may occur after one treatment session, it is generally necessary to perform two to three treatments at least 1 month apart for maximal vessel improvement.

For the treatment of reticular veins or telangiectasias > 1 mm, the long-pulsed Nd:YAG is the laser of choice. Several 1064 nm lasers have the advantage of variable spot sizes and pulse width parameters to treat a wide range of leg veins including small telangiectasias. For superficial vessels < 1 mm in diameter, a 1.5 mm spot, 15–30 ms pulse duration, and 350–600 J/cm^2 is optimal (Lyra; Laserscope, San Jose, CA). For reticular veins measuring 1–4 mm in diameter, a 3–8 mm spot, 30–60 ms pulse duration, and 100–370 J/cm^2 should yield successful results (Lyra; Laserscope, San Jose, CA).

Cooling before, during and after the pulse should always be used to prevent epidermal damage with the use of higher fluences and to increase patient comfort. While the treatment of small-caliber vessels is similar to the KTP, it is useful to apply mild pressure with the

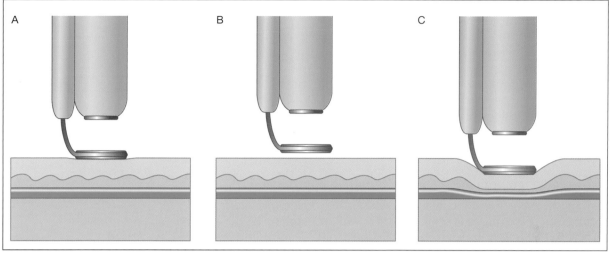

Fig. 6.8 Levels of pressure of the 1064 nm handpiece against the skin. (**A**) The optimal level of pressure is to hold the handpiece gently against the skin with slight pressure. (**B**) Hovering the handpiece above the skin without complete contact may result in inadequate cooling and untoward side effects such as burns or ulceration. (**C**) Pressing too hard with the handpiece may compress the vein, causing inadequate treatment secondary to paucity of the target chromophore hemoglobin

handpiece when treating reticular veins to minimize the diameter and the amount of hemoglobin in the lumen. This will allow greater vessel penetration with less total heat and reduced thermal damage to the surrounding skin. While immediate clearance is often seen with small vessels, larger telangiectasias and reticular veins may yield no visible change during the treatment but should improve over weeks to months.

Swelling, urtication or erythema around treated vessels is common post procedure. The application of ice packs or a topical steroid will speed resolution and lessen the risk of post inflammatory hyperpigmentation. Compression stockings are generally considered unnecessary after the treatment of small telangiectasias. They may improve results when worn for 1 week after the treatment of larger telangiectasias and reticular veins by preventing vessel refilling.

Troubleshooting

In the laser treatment of leg veins, a few common pitfalls exist (Box 6.4). In order to avoid excessive thermal damage, the treating physician must be careful not to re-treat or double pulse vessels when no instantaneous changes are apparent. It can take several minutes after treating an area at appropriate parameters for thermocoagulation to occur.

Retreating an area without allowing the tissue to cool creates excessive thermal injury, which may lead to scarring and ulceration. It is better to work on a separate treatment area and return to the stubborn vessel after 5–10 minutes have passed. Similarly, the lowest

Common pitfalls

- Avoid immediately re-treating or double pulsing vessels when no instantaneous changes are present
- Allow treated areas to cool before attempting a second pass
- Always use the lowest possible effective fluence
- Space adjacent laser pulses at least 1–2 mm apart to reduce excessive thermal damage

Box 6.4 Common pitfalls

possible fluence that will effectively treat a particular vessel should be used to minimize complications. It is always safer to start low and increase to higher energies as needed depending on the vessel response. Blanching of the skin is a sign of excessive thermal injury and should be avoided.

Finally, the physician should be aware of the lateral spread of thermal energy, particularly with the longer wavelength 1064 nm laser. Vessels connected to or adjacent to the treatment pulse area may receive enough thermal damage to effectively coagulate. For this reason, pulses should be separated by at least 1–2 mm.

Side effects, complications, and alternative approaches

Complications of laser therapy for leg veins include epidermal damage, thrombosis, hyperpigmentation, matting, and incomplete clearance (Box 6.5, Fig. 6.9). Patients often find the procedure uncomfortable, but rarely complain of postoperative discomfort. Those who develop telangiectatic matting or incomplete clearance should either undergo re-treatment with the laser or sclerotherapy as appropriate. Localized areas of thrombosis may resolve on their own or can be easily expressed with an 18 gauge needle. Post-procedure hyperpigmentation is generally temporary and the incidence has decreased with the use of longer wavelengths and improved epidermal cooling. As with any laser, meticulous wound care should follow any epidermal damage that occurs to decrease the incidence of scarring. Such wound care may include copious emolliation with a bland petrolatum-based ointment, and crusting and erosions may require a brief course of potent topical steroids.

Side effects
■ Transient hyperpigmentation
■ Purpura
■ Telangiectatic matting
■ Pain
■ Thrombosis
■ Epidermal damage
■ Incomplete clearance

Box 6.5 Side effects

Advanced Topics: Treatment Tips for Experienced Practitioners

1. The monomodal wavelength, varied pulse duration approach is a straightforward, effective method of treatment of leg veins.
2. Wait 8 weeks between treatments with laser technologies.
3. Post-treatment compression is not needed for laser treatment of nonelevated leg veins.
4. Artificial tanners may increase post-inflammatory hyperpigmentation from laser treatment of leg veins.
5. The endpoint of therapy of laser treatment for leg veins is immediate pigment darkening and vasoconstriction.
6. Combined laser/sclerotherapy treatments in a single treatment session may have additive effects.
7. To further reduce the low risk of thrombosis, patients should whenever possible discontinue the use of oral contraceptives prior to receiving laser treatment for leg veins.

Before and After Photographs

See Figures 6.10–6.13 for examples of treatment of reticular leg veins and treatment of spider telangiectasias.

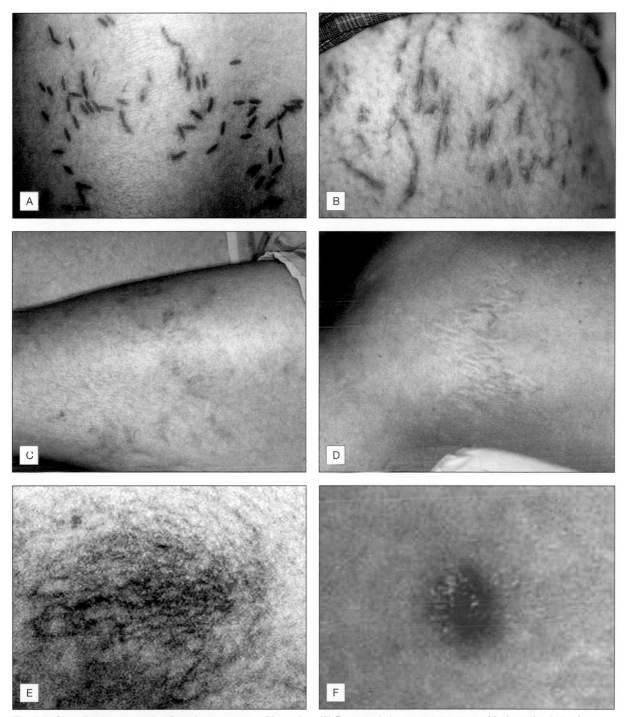

Fig. 6.9 Complications resulting from laser surgery of leg veins. (**A**) Purpura 1 day post-treatment with the pulsed-dye laser (elliptical spot). (**B**) Blisters. (**C**) Transient hyperpigmentation. (**D**) Hypopigmentation occurring in a patient with tanned skin. (**E**) Telangiectatic matting. (**F**) Ulceration

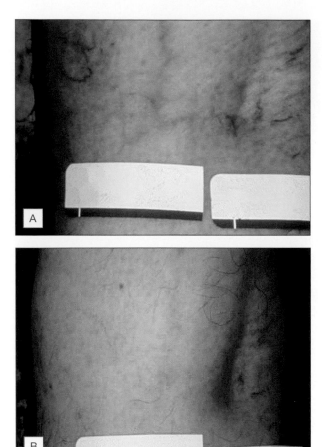

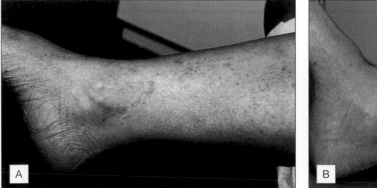

Fig. 6.10 (A) Reticular leg vein pre-treatment. (B) Post-treatment with long pulsed Alexandrite laser 8 mm spot, 70 J/cm^2, 3 ms, three passes (GentleLase, Candela corporation, Wayland, MA) (Photo courtesy of Dr Arielle Kauvar)

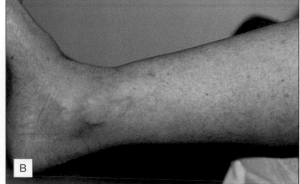

Fig. 6.11 (A) Reticular leg vein pre-treatment. (B) Post-treatment with long-pulsed 1064 nm laser (Courtesy of Dr Thomas E. Rohrer)

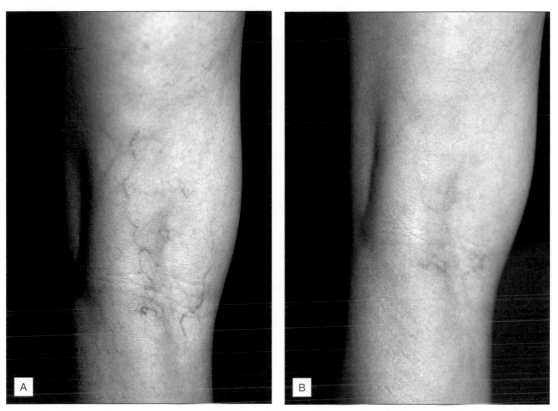

Fig. 6.12 (**A**) Larger leg telangiectasia pre-treatment. (**B**) Post-treatment with pulsed dye laser 3×10 mm elliptical spot, 10 ms, 18 J/cm^2, 50/20 DCD (Vbeam, Candela corporation, Wayland, MA) (Photos courtesy of Dr Thomas E. Rohrer)

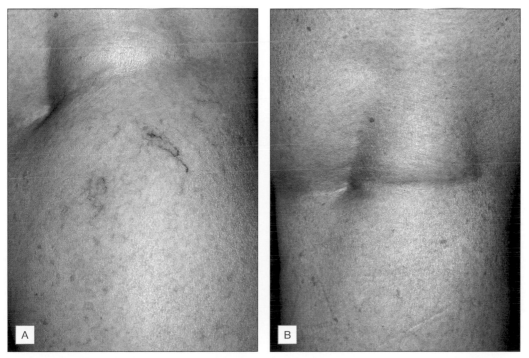

Fig. 6.13 (**A**) Spider telangiectasias pre-treatment. (**B**) Post three treatments at 8-week intervals with the long-pulsed 1064 nm laser (Courtesy of Dr Thomas E. Rohrer)

Further Reading

Bernstein EF 2001 Clinical characteristics of 500 consecutive patients presenting for laser removal of lower extremity spider veins. Dermatologic Surgery 27:31–33

Dover JS, Sadick NS, Goldman MP 1999 The role of lasers and light sources in the treatment of leg veins. Dermatologic Surgery 25:328–336

Eremia S, Li C, Umar SH 2002 A side-by-side comparative study of 1,064 nm Nd:Yag, 810 nm diode and 755 nm alexandrite for treatment of 0.3–3 mm leg veins. Dermatologic Surgery 28:224–230

Kauvar AN 2000 The role of lasers in the treatment of leg veins. Seminars in Cutaneous Medicine and Surgery 19:245–252

Levy JL, Elbahr C, Jouve E, Mordon S 2004 Comparison and sequential study of long pulsed Nd:Yag 1,064 nm laser and sclerotherapy in leg telangiectasias treatment. Lasers in Surgery and Medicine 34:273–276

Omura NE, Dover JS, Arndt KA, Kauvar AN 2003 Treatment of reticular leg veins with a 1064 nm long-pulsed Nd:Yag laser. Journal of the American Academy of Dermatology 48:76–81

Ross EV, Domankevitz Y 2003 Laser leg vein treatment: a brief overview. Journal of Cosmetic and Laser Therapy 5:192–197

Sadick NS 2003 Laser treatment with a 1064 nm laser for lower extremity class I–III veins employing variable spots and pulse width parameters. Dermatologic Surgery 29:916–919

Sadick NS, Makino Y 2004 Selective electro-thermolysis in aesthetic medicine: a review. Lasers in Surgery and Medicine 34:91–97

Sadick NS, Trelles MA 2005 A clinical, histological, and computer-based assessment of the Polaris LV, combination diode and radiofrequency system, for leg vein treatment. Lasers in Surgery and Medicine 36:98–104

Sadick NS, Weiss RA, Goldman MP 2002 Advances in laser surgery for leg veins: bimodal wavelength approach to lower extremity vessels, new cooling techniques, and longer pulse durations. Dermatologic Surgery 28:16–20

7

Ambulatory Phlebectomy

Albert-Adrien Ramelet

Introduction

Already described in Roman times and in Middle Ages, and rediscovered by the Swiss dermatologist Robert Muller, ambulatory phlebectomy (AP) is a safe and effective surgical technique that enables the removal of incompetent saphenous veins (except the saphenofemoral and in most cases the saphenopopliteal junctions), their major tributaries, perforators, and reticular veins, including the feeding veins of telangiectasias, or even blue telangiectasias. Ambulatory phlebectomy may also be used in varicophlebitis and superficial phlebitis, or for veins in other locations, for instance dilated periorbital, temporal or frontal venous networks, as well as venous dilatation of the abdomen, arms or dorsum of the hands.

AP is indicated in almost all patients, including the elderly. Most of the procedures are performed in truly ambulatory patients, but the technique may also be used in conjunction with other surgical procedures in ambulatory or stationary patients.

The goal of ambulatory phlebectomy is to secure definitive treatment of the varicose veins, once the underlying cause of reflux has been treated and eliminated. In some cases, the goal may be only partial or short-term improvement. Examples include avulsion of a single painful varicose vein in a young mother unwilling or unable to consider more extensive treatment, or in an elderly patient, removal of a single symptomatic varicose segment or of a feeding vein causing a leg ulcer.

The problem being treated

This chapter will clarify how to select patients who may benefit from AP and how to safely and effectively perform the procedure. However, AP cannot be learned solely from a textbook, and being able to perform the procedure independently requires observing an experienced phlebologist treat different kinds of varicose veins as he or she carefully explains the successive steps of infusing anesthesia, operating and bandaging.

Every patient should be carefully interviewed and examined, with the examination including at least a hand-held Doppler, but preferably duplex ultrasound (DUS), before selection of the most appropriate procedure (Box 7.1). Transillumination is a useful tool for detecting reticular varicose veins and feeding veins associated with overlying telangiectasias.

Patient Selection

Patients of all ages may be treated with AP. All types of primary or secondary varicose veins (saphenous, reticular, perineal, telangiectatic, and perforating veins corresponding to classes C_1–C_6 of the clinical, etiologic, anatomic, pathophysiologic classification (CEAP)) may be removed by AP (Boxes 7.2, 7.3; Figs 7.1–7.3). Further special indications are discussed at the end of this chapter.

Regional venous networks particularly appropriate for ambulatory phlebectomy include accessory saphenous veins of the thigh, groin pudendal veins, reticular varicose veins (popliteal fossa, lateral thigh and leg, as described by Albanese), veins of the ankles, and the dorsal venous network of the foot.

While most procedures are performed in ambulatory patients, the technique may also be used in conjunction with other surgical procedures such as high ligations (crossectomy) and stripping of incompetent saphenous veins in ambulatory or stationary patients.

Contraindications are rare or relative: critical arterial ischemia, infections, allergy to local anesthetics, bed-ridden status, and impaired blood clotting or immunity. AP is usually not performed during pregnancy or immediately postpartum, as varicose veins frequently regress spontaneously.

Diagnostic methods

- Patient interview
- Clinical examination while the patient is in the supine position
- Transillumination
- Doppler or duplex ultrasound

Box 7.1 Diagnostic methods

Indications for AP

- Saphenous and saphenous collateral varicose veins
- Reticular varicose veins
- Perineal varicose veins
- Veins of the dorsal aspect of the foot
- Varicose pearls
- Perforators (with some limits)

Phlebectomy of an isolated portion of a saphenous vein should not be conducted if the termination is insufficient. Phlebectomy of the perforators is to be envisaged with caution. The results are good if the hook is used to remove the medial perforators of the thigh and small perforators of the lateral surface of the legs. The results are mediocre with respect to the medial perforators of the lower leg

Other indications
- Curettage of telangiectasias

Other esthetic indications
- Facial, palpebral and arm veins, etc.

Box 7.3 Indications for AP

C classes in CEAP (2004)

C_0: No visible or palpable signs of venous disease
C_1: Telangiectasias or reticular veins
C_2: Varicose veins; distinguished from reticular veins by a diameter of 3 mm or more
C_3: Edema
C_4: Changes in skin and subcutaneous tissue secondary to chronic venous disorders (CVD)
C_{4a}: Pigmentation or eczema
C_{4b}: Lipodermatosclerosis or atrophie blanche
C_5: Healed venous ulcer
C_6: Active venous ulcer

Each clinical class is further characterized by a subscript for the presence of symptoms (S = symptomatic) or absence of symptoms (A = asymptomatic). Symptoms include aching, pain, tightness, skin irritation, heaviness, muscle cramps, and other complaints attributable to venous dysfunction. (Adapted from Eklof B, et al 2004 Revision of the CEAP classification for chronic venous disorders: consensus statement. Journal of Vascular Surgery 40:1248–1252)

Box 7.2 C classes in CEAP (2004)

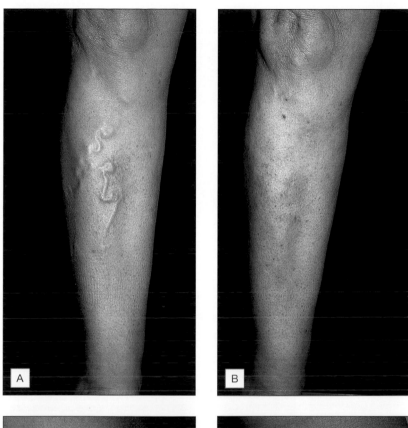

Fig. 7.1 (**A**) Pretibial varicose veins (C2). (**B**) 6 weeks after AP

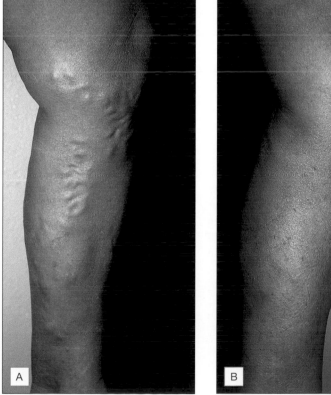

Fig. 7.2 (**A**) Saphenous accessory varicose veins, incompetence of Dodd's perforator (C2). (**B**) 6 weeks after AP

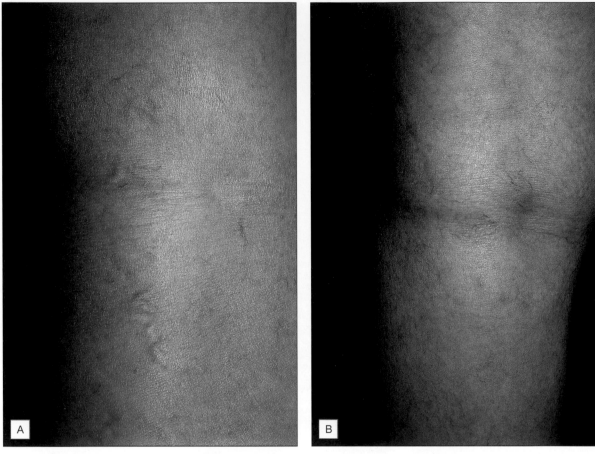

Fig. 7.3 (A) Reticular varicose veins (C1). **(B)** 6 weeks after AP

Expected Benefits

Since Muller's first writings in 1966, AP has been considered a very effective and economical technique that affords outstanding cosmetic results.

Long-term results tend to be excellent as long as the most proximal source of reflux is eliminated, however evidence-based objective data confirming this widely accepted conclusion continue to be sparse. A single randomized, controlled trial by de Ross has recently been published and found excellent long-term results of AP and verified its superiority to sclerotherapy for treatment of the lateral accessory vein of the thigh.

Improvement in anesthetic technique with the advent of tumescence has resulted in greatly reduced pre- and postoperative pain as well as complications. As AP is usually performed in the friendly environment of an office rather than in the operating room, it is mostly experienced as 'quite comfortable' by patients.

The technique is safe, as noted by several publications that have reviewed reported complications of AP. The side effects of this procedure will be discussed further later.

It should be noted that in order to obtain good results and prevent recurrences, AP must only be performed when it is indicated. When this procedure is selected, it must consist of removal of all segments of varicose veins, including feeding perforators, to prevent relapses or unsightly complications, such as telangiectatic matting.

AP is an easy and inexpensive procedure to perform. A skilled practitioner may remove an extensive array of varicose veins in a short period of time, generally lasting 20–90 minutes, with both legs being operated upon in a single session. A simple, streamlined operative approach by a well-trained practitioner is much more effective and economical than 'high-tech' new modalities.

Sclerotherapy may initially appear to be even easier to perform and more economical than AP, but for veins larger than superficial telangiectasias, the number of sessions are required and the high rate of recurrence excludes this option (Box 7.4).

Overview of Treatment Strategy

Treatment approach and major determinants

Major treatment modalities in phlebology include compression therapy, sclerotherapy, AP, surgery, and laser treatment. Each technique has its own indications and advantages, although there are some areas of overlap.

For most indications, the procedure most similar to AP is sclerotherapy. Sclerotherapy is principally indicated in the treatment of telangiectasias and reticular varicose veins. New modalities, such as foam sclerotherapy and ultrasound-guided sclerotherapy, afford excellent results in the treatment of intrafascial varicose networks, including the lesser saphenous veins, or saphenous and accessory saphenous veins of the thigh.

AP is superior to sclerotherapy in the treatment of medium to large, epifascial varicose veins. With AP, there are fewer recurrences, and no risks of inadvertent intra-arterial injection, skin necrosis (due to extravasation of sclerosant or unpredictable arteriovenous anastomosis injection), or residual hyperpigmentation.

Patient Interviews

Elicitation of patient histories is discussed in a previous chapter. Recording of structured case histories permits appropriate weighting of the various symptoms and venous risk factors, and improved estimation of prognosis.

The physician must be especially receptive to the patient's complaints and expectations, as postoperative patient disappointment is often less a matter of technical failure than the result of unrealistic patient expectations that were unchallenged prior to treatment.

Careful analysis of the patient's history and symptoms may enable the physician to differentiate venous problems from arterial lesions, nerve root irritation syndrome, osteoarticular or muscle-tendon disease, and more generalized diseases such as fibromyalgia. Some symptoms, such as muscle cramps and restless legs, are not very specific.

Principal indications of sclerotherapy and AP[a]

- **Sclerotherapy**: telangiectasias and reticular varicose veins
- **Ultrasound-guided sclerotherapy**: intrafascial varicose networks, including the lesser saphenous veins
- **Ambulatory phlebectomy**: from reticular to large, epifascial varicose veins

[a]These indications are debatable. The choice of the method depends first on the skill of the practitioner and local traditions.

Box 7.4 Principal indications of sclerotherapy and AP[a]

Treatment of varicose veins is unlikely to result in the resolution of these symptoms, and the patient should be made aware of this.

The prognosis and likely evolution of chronic venous disease in each particular patient should also be discussed. Depending on the predominant type of varicose veins, the severity of the disorder, and presence of specific risk factors, patients may be likely to encounter different clinical courses in the future.

Clinical Examination

This is an essential part of the treatment, as good AP results depend on the accuracy of the diagnosis and of a thorough evaluation of the exact origin and extent of the varicose veins. Clinical examination should be supplemented by Doppler and/or duplex ultrasound, as described in Chapter 3 (Box 7.1).

Treatment Techniques

Equipment

Only a few surgical instruments and forms of equipment are required (Box 7.5) for AP. Among the types of hooks that have been marketed for vein grasping and extraction are the Müller, Oesch, Ramelet, Tretbar, and Varady (Figs 7.4–7.7).

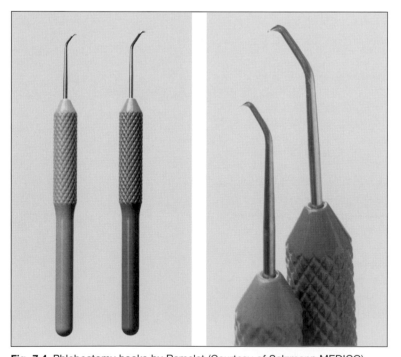

Fig. 7.4 Phlebectomy hooks by Ramelet (Courtesy of Salzmann MEDICO)

Equipment necessary for phlebectomy

- Local buffered anesthetic, normal saline or Ringer's solution
- Resuscitation equipment, indispensable during any procedure
- Sterile gloves and mask
- Disinfectant (not removing the marking stain of the course of varicose veins)
- No. 11 straight blade scalpel
- 18 gauge needle
- Phlebectomy hooks
- Mosquito forceps
- Sterile pads
- Dressing materials
- Elastic bandages

Box 7.5 Equipment necessary for phlebectomy

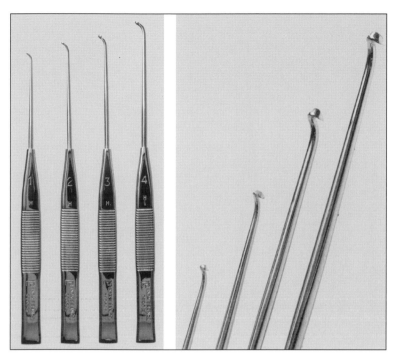

Fig. 7.5 Phlebectomy hooks by Müller (Courtesy of Salzmann MEDICO)

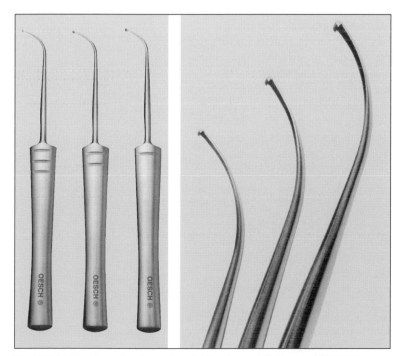

Fig. 7.6 Phlebectomy hooks by Oesch (Courtesy of Salzmann MEDICO)

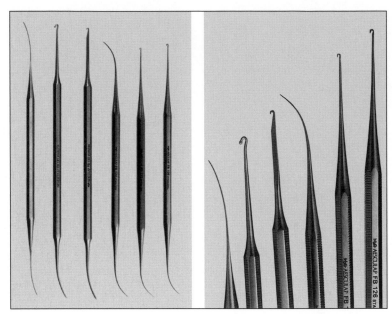

Fig. 7.7 Phlebectomy hooks by Varady (Courtesy of Salzmann MEDICO)

Blunt hooks should not be used as successful hooks must pass under the vein in order to pull it out, with the skin incision as long as the diameter of the curvature of the hook. Some also suggest the use of a dissector to release the vein. Its value is highly debatable as the associated incisions tend to be wider, with a higher risk of visible scars.

The Ramelet hook (comes in two sizes) has some particular advantages (Fig. 7.5). The cylindrical grip permits gentle rolling of the hook between the fingers, thus diminishing the amount of rotation of the wrists and minimizing wrist and hand stress during the procedure. The shaft is short and allows precise and close work as well as moderate traction. The hook's angulation facilitates vein dissection, while the sharp tip grips the perivenous collagen bundles and tunica externa of the veins, allowing these to be lifted from above. In this manner, damage to the surrounding tissues and lymphatics is limited. The sharp tip is also useful for the curettage of telangiectasias (see later).

Treatment algorithm

Before the procedure, the patient should receive instructions explaining the technique, and likely results and risks. Shaving or otherwise depilating the leg before the operation is required. Premedication is seldom needed and generally should be avoided as it limits postoperative ambulation, which is an important strategy for preventing thromboembolic complications.

Marking of varicose veins

Examination of the patient and marking (with a KMnO4 or felt tip pen for epidiascope) of the target veins prior to beginning the treatment is an essential step. Marking should be performed while the patient is in a standing and supine position, as some varicosities, in particular reticular veins, are more visible when the patient is lying down. Mapping veins by using transillumination significantly enhances the technique of AP by permitting more accurate visualization of the course of a varicose vein prior to extraction (Fig. 7.8). Marking may also be facilitated by echography to detect nonpalpable venous networks between the visible varicosities (Fig. 7.9).

Local anesthesia

After a thorough disinfection of the leg (taking care not to erase preoperative marking), local anesthesia consisting of buffered Lidocaine with epinephrine diluted in saline or Ringer's solution (Figs 7.10, 7.11) is infused using the tumescent technique (Box 7.6). Tumescence anesthesia has numerous advantages: (1) virtually painless injection; (2) a low risk of toxicity even during very extensive bilateral phlebectomies; (3) hydrodissection of the vein by paravascular injection;

Tumescence local anesthesia (Klein's Formula, modified)

- Lidocaine (1%)–epinephrine: 50 ml
- 8.4% sodium bicarbonate: 5 ml
- Normal saline or Ringer's solution 500 ml

Box 7.6 Tumescence local anesthesia (Klein's formula, modified)

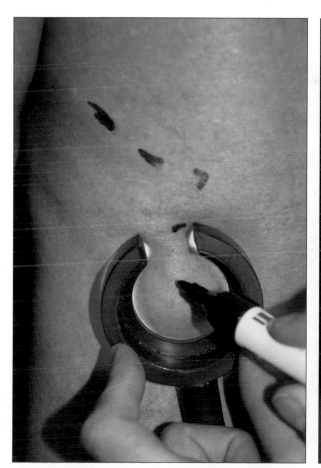

Fig. 7.8 Transillumination mapping. Invisible superficial varicose veins are easily detected with transillumination (VeinLite; courtesy of Wagner Medical)

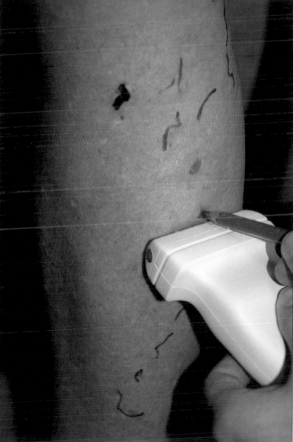

Fig. 7.9 Echo-guided marking using echography to detect nonpalpable venous network between the varicosities

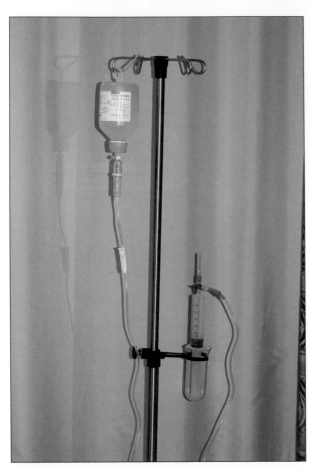

Fig. 7.10 Tumescent anesthesia: three-way system with buffered Lidocaine–epinephrine diluted in saline or Ringer's solution

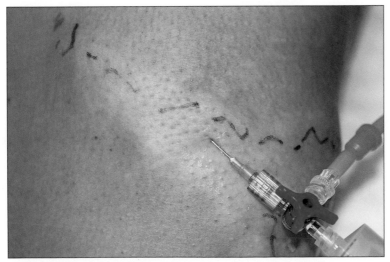

Fig. 7.11 Tumescent anesthesia: tumescent infiltration of the varicose network

(4) compression of engorged neighboring tissues that decreases bleeding and prevents hematomas; (5) 'rinsing' of any blood collection as the solution drips out through incisions during the hours following the operation; and (6) a prolonged analgesic effect.

Preoperative sclerotherapy

This can reduce telangiectasias and ensures a better immediate cosmetic result. Sclerotherapy should be performed before the start of the AP operation, as telangiectasias become less visible after injection of tumescent anesthesia.

Operation

Skin incisions made with the point of the scalpel (Fig. 7.12) or using a needle (Fig. 7.13) are oriented vertically (thigh, leg) or along lines of minimal skin tension (knee, ankles). The interval between the

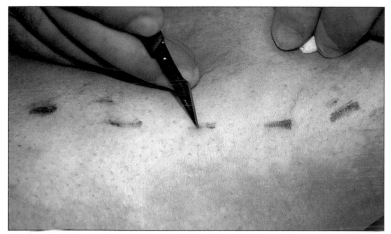

Fig. 7.12 Scalpel tip incision

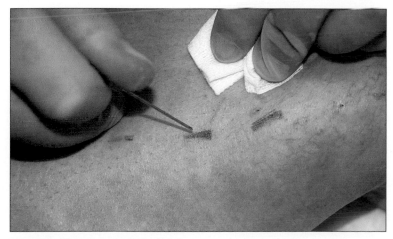

Fig. 7.13 18 gauge needle tip incision

incisions varies according to the size and character of the varicose vein to be treated. Once the varicosity is dissected and grasped with the hook (Figs 7.14, 7.15), it is detached from its fibroadipose bed and extracted using mosquito forceps held in the left hand (Figs 7.16–7.18). Its entire course is removed by sliding the divided incompetent vein from one incision to the other. Neither venous ligation nor sutures of the skin are required. Perforators are extirpated by gentle and regular traction.

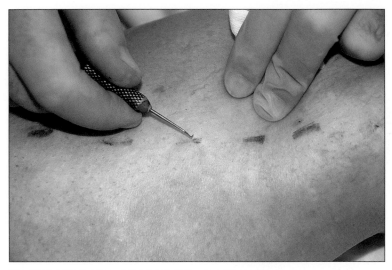

Fig. 7.14 Introduction of the hook through a tiny incision

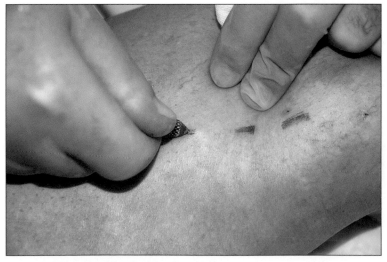

Fig. 7.15 Dissection of varicose vein using hook

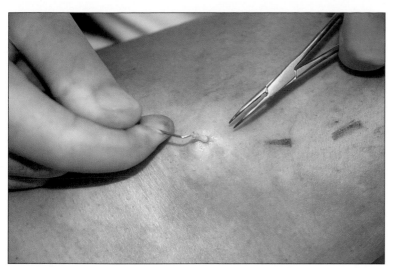

Fig. 7.16 Extraction of varicose vein on tip of hook; the operator's left hand is holding mosquito forceps, ready to grasp the varicose vein

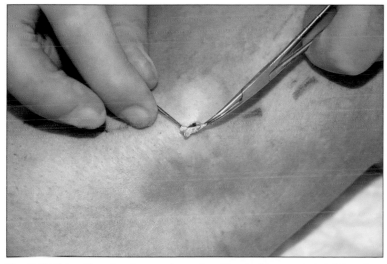

Fig. 7.17 Extraction of varicose vein on tip of hook; the operator's left hand has grasped the varicose vein with the mosquito forceps

Hemostasis is secured by compressing the bleeding point with the left hand or by an assistant in difficult cases. Regions where hemostasis is difficult to achieve (in the thigh, popliteal fossa, dorsum of the foot, or greatly dilated perforators) are treated first.

Dressing

After cleaning the leg with hydrogen peroxide, absorbent sterile dressings are applied to the incisions and covered by a tubular knit stocking

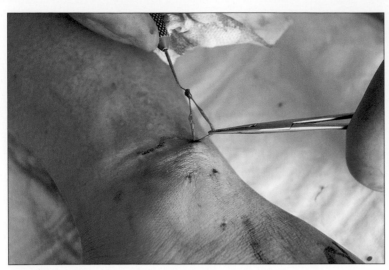

Fig. 7.18 Extraction of varicose vein using hook and mosquito forceps. The varicosity is then freed stepwise, from one incision to the other

(Fig. 7.19). Compression is provided by a robust elastic bandage, applied from the toe joints and extending up proximally to the operated areas (Fig. 7.20). Immediate postoperative application of compression hosieries or another type of bandage is an alternative.

Postoperative pain is rare. Prophylactic anticoagulation is not indicated as the patient moves during the operation and walks immediately afterwards with a compression bandage.

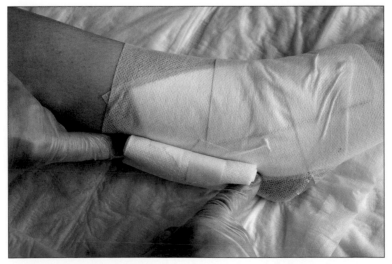

Fig. 7.19 Application of an absorbent dressing, held in place by adhesives and covered by a tubular knit stocking

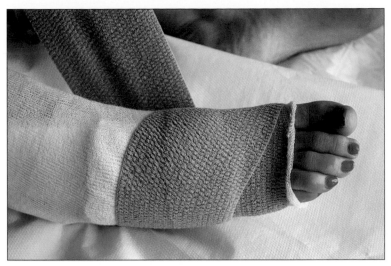

Fig. 7.20 A robust elastic bandage is applied from the toe joints, extending up proximally to the operated areas

Selective compression is justified when there is a notable risk of bleeding. Rolled pads are applied along the course of the varicose vein, which has been removed. The malleoli, retromalleolar gutters and popliteal fossa may be protected by placing packing (cotton balls) before the bandage is applied.

The dressing should be very tight after the procedure, loosened for the night, and retightened the next morning.

Postoperative Course

A postoperative instruction sheet to be distributed to the patient is a valuable tool (Box 7.7). The following guidelines should be given to the patient:

1. The patient must walk immediately after the procedure and immediate return to everyday activities and normal life is indicated.
2. It is preferable to avoid driving a vehicle on the day of the procedure due to the risks of anxiety and disorientation, transitory paresis of the foot due to anesthesia of deep nerves, and exceptional cases of postoperative faintness. No time off work is usually required.
3. Postoperative pain is minimal, especially with tumescent anesthesia.
4. The dressing is changed after 48 hours (Fig. 7.21). From then on, bandages or Class II compression stockings are worn only from the morning to the night for 3 weeks.
5. Short showers are permitted starting from the fourth day after the procedure.
6. Sun exposure has to be avoided until the fine erythematous marks have faded.
7. Results are usually quite impressive a few weeks after the procedure (Fig. 7.22).

Postoperative instruction sheet for patients

Postoperative instructions

Ambulatory phlebectomy is a minor operation that is very well tolerated. It takes place in the doctor's office. Only the path of the sick vein is anesthetized (injections along the varicose vein). The procedure consists of removing the varicose vein through small incisions, leaving very discreet scars after a few months. Sick and useless veins that have been removed cannot recur but it is of course possible that you will subsequently develop other varicose veins independent of the current treatment. Those varicose veins can also be removed surgically if necessary. The operation takes place in an outpatient setting and no sick leave or interruption of everyday life is necessary.

On the day of the operation, remember to:

■ Shave or depilate all of the leg a few days before surgery
■ Take a last bath or shower just before the procedure, since you will not be able to wet the leg (or legs) for 4 days
■ Do not apply cream or ointment to the legs the day before or the morning of the operation
■ Wear sufficiently wide shoes: the bandage begins at the root of the toes, where it will be tightest
■ In certain cases, underwear may be stained during disinfection. If appropriate, wear easily washed underwear and bring replacement underwear
■ It is not advisable to drive after the procedure. It is preferable to have somebody drive you or take public transport
■ Lastly, arrive relaxed since the local anesthesia and procedure are very well tolerated. It is preferable to eat breakfast before you come

After the procedure:

■ It is important for you to walk and move around a lot after the operation and over the following days. This is the best (and most natural) way of preventing venous complications, which are exceptional with this technique
■ The bandages will be worn day and night for 48 hours after the operation. **You should loosen the bandages at night and tighten them in the morning**
■ After 24 or 48 hours, the dressing will be changed in the doctor's office
■ You will then wear bandages or varicose vein stockings during the day, only from getting up to going to bed, for 20 days. It is essential to wear the elastic compression (varicose vein stockings or stretch-bandages). At night, simply raise your legs (blocks under the feet of the bed, etc.)
■ A short shower is authorized on postoperative day 4.

Box 7.7 Postoperative instruction sheet for patients

Troubleshooting

Technical difficulties are related to: (1) the size of the varicose veins, with fine reticular varicose veins being particularly troublesome; (2) the veins' strength and morphology, including the presence of fibrosis and attachment to neighboring tissues in case of previous thrombophlebitis or sclerotherapy, and of unusual fragility in the elderly; (3) the location of the incompetent vein, with challenging surfaces being the medial surface of the thigh, popliteal fossa, prepatellar area, and ankle and dorsum of the foot); and (4) patient obesity, especially wide thigh girth.

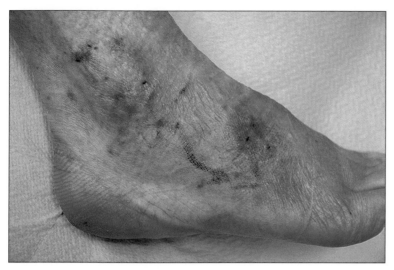

Fig. 7.21 Aspect 48 hours after the procedure, when changing the dressing. Hematomas are quite discrete

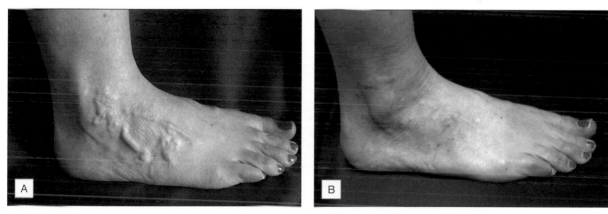

Fig. 7.22 (**A**) Dorsal network of the foot, preoperative appearance. (**B**) 6 weeks after the procedure

Success in such challenging conditions requires good training, prior experience, and meticulous attention to every clinical and technical detail.

Side Effects

Inappropriate patient selection leads to poor results with postoperative recurrences soon after treatment, or emergence of so-called neo-telangiectasias (telangiectatic matting). The latter problem is particularly likely if proximal venous reflux has not been corrected.

Insufficient skill in surgery or in compression causes hematomas, bandage-induced edema, scars and matting.

Hemorrhage, hematomas, transient hyperpigmentation, or transient slight matting are not uncommon and should be considered undesirable but routine postoperative events rather than true complications.

Complications

These are mostly benign and resolve spontaneously (Box 7.8).

Neo-telangiectasias (telangiectatis matting) disappearing on pressure under glass are not rare after phlebectomy, stripping or sclerotherapy. Such matting may spontaneously remit after a few months or persist. Further sclerotherapy or laser treatment may help matting fade. In some cases matting is due to the continued presence of a nearby small perforator, which may be removed with phlebectomy. While telangiectatic matting is not rare, it is quite troublesome as the aim of phlebectomy is often to improve cosmetic appearance.

Other complications include lymphatic pseudocysts (occurring mainly at the ankle, pretibial or popliteal areas), and temporary or definitive dysesthesia and nerve damage. Wound infection, keloid formation, Koebner phenomenon (psoriasis, lichen planus, and vitiligo), tattooing, phlebitis, and deep vein thrombosis, are rare complications.

Occasional complications of AP

Cutaneous
- Blisters
- Hyper- or hypopigmentation
- Local infection
- Visible scars
- Exceptional complications: tattooing, skin necrosis, silicotic granuloma due to application of talc, Koebner's phenomenon (psoriasis, vitiligo or lichen planus, etc.)

Vascular
- Postoperative bleeding
- Hematomas
- Neotelangiectasias (matting)
- Lymphatic pseudocyst, lymphorrhea
- Postoperative edema (dorsum of the foot)
- Superficial phlebitis
- Deep vein thrombosis

Neurological
- Transient or definitive damage to sensory nerves
- Tarsus syndrome consecutive to unadapted compression
- Neuromas

General
- Faintness
- Allergy to anesthetics

Box 7.8 Occasional complications of AP

After phlebectomy of the dorsum of the foot, postoperative edema may persist for several weeks.

Malaise resulting from local anesthesia or vasovagal reaction is no longer observed since the introduction of the tumescent technique. Allergy to the anesthetic is extremely rare. It may occur as true Lidocaine allergy or as the result of allergy to preservatives (parabens group), commonly present in multiple dose vials. Resuscitation equipment, including oxygen, and personnel trained in advanced resuscitation techniques must always be available, if necessary (Box 7.9).

As with any therapeutic procedure, the patient has to be warned about poor results and potential complications; this is particularly important when the aim of the treatment is cosmetic improvement.

Alternative Methods

Failure of the procedure may occur, especially when the vein is located deeply in the subcutaneous or intrafascial space, is extremely small, or associated with an area of prior inflammation.

When AP is not feasible, the primary alternative treatment is sclerotherapy, including that with ultrasound guidance. Sclerotherapy is also indicated if the patient is reluctant to undergo surgery.

Special Indications

Curettage of telangiectasias

The treatment of telangiectasias may be quite disappointing. Feeding veins should be removed by AP or treated with sclerotherapy in order to diminish the risk of recurrence of telangiectasias. Unfortunately, feeding veins are not always easily detectable and transillumination may be needed to identify them. Larger telangiectasias may be destroyed by gentle subcutaneous curettage with the sharp harpoon of the blue Ramelet's hook (Fig. 7.23), with the resulting debris being removed through tiny incisions. This technique is not yet in widespread use, but an experienced phlebologist may achieve quite good results, even in difficult cases.

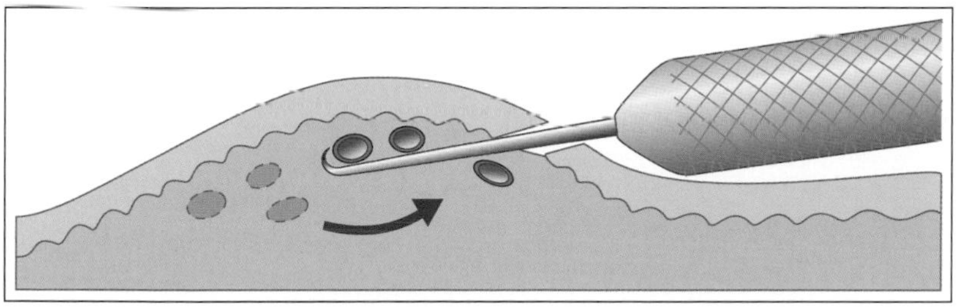

Key components of resuscitation equipment

- Epinephrine
- Diphenhydramine
- Solumedrol
- Diazepam
- Intubation kit[a]
- Oxygen
- Ambu bag
- Ringer's or saline solution
- Defibrillator[a]

[a]The interest of these devices in an office is debatable. They are useless if the practitioner has not been well trained in resuscitation. Note also that this list varies according to local customs, distance to emergency rooms, etc. and it should not be forgotten that accidents are merely inexistent when performing AP in one office. It is more important to know whom to call in case of emergency!

Box 7.9 Key components of resuscitation equipment

Fig. 7.23 Curettage of telangiectasias with Ramelet's blue hook

Superficial thrombophlebitis

Phlebectomy can also be used as an immediate treatment for small segments of superficial thrombophlebitis. The intravascular coagulum is expressed (Fig. 7.24) and the involved vein segment can be extracted through the same incision. The patient is very rapidly relieved of discomfort and the underlying vein is eliminated in one step.

Debatable New Developments of the Technique

Echo-guided phlebectomy

Relatively inaccessible varicose veins (mainly at the thigh) may be removed with a hook under ultrasonographic control. This is similar in principle to the technique of echo-guided sclerotherapy.

Transillumination-powered phlebectomy

Varicose veins are resected after aspiration and invagination into a disposable cannula within which rotates a cylindrical shaver. This technique is based on use of a sophisticated device that requires expensive disposable accessories. Side effects appear to be common and the promise of this technique remains to be realized.

Veins in other locations

Ambulatory phlebectomy of anatomical regions other than the legs is possible. Dilated periorbital, temporal or frontal venous networks may be treated. AP of venous dilatation of the abdomen (if the veins in

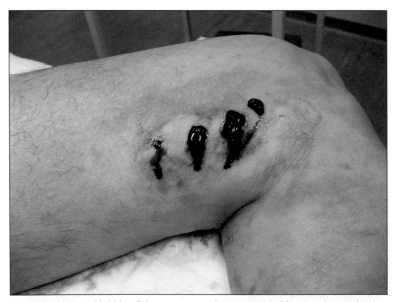

Fig. 7.24 Varicophlebitis of the greater saphenous vein. After local anesthesia, the incision allows expression of the thrombus. In the case of fresh varicophlebitis, phlebectomy of the varicose vein may be combined with thrombectomy

question are not directly associated with a deep venous obstruction) may also be performed. Finally, dilated veins of the arms, dorsum of the hands, or penis may also be removed with AP. However, removal of functional veins for purely esthetic reasons remains controversial.

Other uses of hook technique

Ramelet's hook has also been used to remove implanted drug delivery systems, such as Norplant, with minimal scarring. Vein biopsy may also be performed using this simple device.

Further reading

Olivencia JA 2000 Complications of ambulatory phlebectomy: a review of 4000 consecutive cases. American Journal of Cosmetic Surgery 17:161–165

Olivencia JA 2003 Minimally invasive vein surgery. Techniques in Vascular Interventional Radiology 6:121–124

Olivencia JA 2004 Ambulatory phlebectomy turned 2400 years old. Dermatologic Surgery 30:704–708

Ramelet AA 1997 Complications of ambulatory phlebectomy. Dermatologic Surgery 23:947–954

Ramelet AA 1999 Télangiectasie: indications de la phlébectomie. Acta Médecine Interne et Angiologie 15:38–42

Ramelet AA 2002 Phlebectomy – cosmetic indications. Journal of Cosmetic Dermatology 1:13–19

Ramelet AA 2004 La phlébectomie selon Muller, description de la technique sous sa forme actuelle. Phlébologie 57:309–317

Roos KP de, Nieman FHM, Neumann HAM 2003 Ambulatory phlebectomy versus compression therapy: results of a randomized controlled trial. Dermatologic Surgery 29:221–226

Weiss RA, Ramelet AA 2002 Varicose veins treated with ambulatory phlebectomy. Emedecine Journal 3:748 http://www.emedicine.com/derm/topic748.htm

Weiss RA, Ramelet AA 2002 Removal of blue periocular lower eyelid veins by ambulatory phlebectomy. Dermatologic Surgery 28:43–45

8

Endovenous Ablation

Steven E. Zimmet

Introduction

The problem being treated

This chapter will present use of endovenous techniques, namely endovenous laser ablation (EVLA) and radiofrequency ablation (RFA, Closure, VNUS Medical Technologies Inc., San Jose, CA) to treat greater saphenous vein (GSV) incompetence. These methods involve delivering either laser or radiofrequency energy endovenously to cause fibrotic occlusion of a vein.

Underlying GSV incompetence is common in the approximately 25% of women and 15% of men who have lower extremity venous insufficiency. The GSV runs from the medial ankle to the groin, where it empties into the femoral vein at the saphenofemoral junction (SFJ). Note that other underlying veins, such as the small saphenous vein (SSV), perforators, accessory saphenous veins and pudendal veins may be the source of surface varices.

This chapter will not cover duplex ultrasound (DUS) examination, an essential tool in endovenous ablation. DUS is used to: (1) delineate the pattern of underlying incompetence; (2) map the GSV; (3) guide percutaneous access for placement of the sheath and laser fiber/radiofrequency catheter; (4) monitor delivery of tumescent anesthesia; and (5) assess results at follow up. Other topics that will not be covered include elicitation of a complete history and physical examination, and concurrent provision of ancillary treatments, such as routine sclerotherapy, foam sclerotherapy, ultrasound-guided sclerotherapy and ambulatory phlebectomy. Information regarding these techniques is available in other chapters.

Patient Selection (Box 8.1)

Indications for endovenous treatment include GSV reflux in an ambulatory patient who has surface varices and/or symptoms or complications related to superficial venous insufficiency. Typical symptoms include restless legs, leg aching, heaviness, fatigue, night cramps, and pruritus. Complications of superficial venous insufficiency include venous thromboembolism, edema, eczema, lipodermatosclerosis, venous ulceration, and spontaneous hemorrhage. Ablation of reflux, whether

---

Patient selection for endovenous ablation

- Ambulatory patient without contraindications
- Those with the following signs: bulging varicose veins with or without signs of chronic venous insufficiency (edema, dermatitis, pigmentation of the lower leg, lipodermatosclerosis, venous ulceration, spontaneous hemorrhage)
- Those with the following symptoms: leg heaviness, aching, fatigue, night cramps, pruritus, restless leg syndrome)
- Ultrasound findings: incompetence of the GSV. The GSV should have minimal tortuosity so as to permit appropriate placement of the sheath and catheter/fiber

Box 8.1 Patient selection for endovenous ablation

accomplished with surgical, sclerotherapy or endovenous techniques, improves symptoms and stigmata of chronic venous insufficiency.

The contraindications to endovenous treatment are listed in Box 8.2.

Expected Benefits: General

Endovenous procedures are less invasive alternatives compared with stripping. They may be performed using local anesthesia, with or without supplemental oral anxiolytics, and are comfortable for the patient in an office setting. EVLA generally takes between 30–60 minutes, while RFA requires about 45–75 minutes. Procedure times are dependent on the length of segment treated, experience of the operator and whether ancillary procedures, such as ambulatory phlebectomy, are carried out. Patient satisfaction has been reported to be very high following both procedures.

The outcomes following endovenous treatment include total occlusion of the treated segment, early failure (complete or segmental), or late recanalization (complete or segmental). The GSV is often sonographically absent 1 year post-treatment.

Regardless of how underlying saphenous incompetence is treated, ancillary treatments are generally needed to treat residual varices. Such treatments may include cutaneous laser, sclerotherapy (liquid and/or foam), and ambulatory phlebectomy (Fig. 8.1).

CPT codes and physician payment rates have recently been established for EVLA and RFA (Box 8.3).

Expected Benefits: Radiofrequency Ablation

RF catheters generate heat slowly in a zone around the tissue–electrode interface. Feedback-controlled heating of the vein to 85–90°C causes endothelial destruction, collagen contraction, and vein wall thickening, collectively resulting in vein occlusion. Good contact between the electrodes and vein wall is essential. The manufacturer

Contraindications to endovenous procedures

- Active implanted device: consult the cardiologist and the manufacturer prior to doing radiofrequency ablation
- Allergy to local anesthetic
- Hypercoagulable states
- Infection of the leg to be treated
- Lymphedema
- Nonambulatory patient
- Peripheral arterial insufficiency
- Poor general health
- Pregnancy
- Recent/active venous thromboembolism
- Thrombus or synechiae in the vein to be treated
- Tortuous GSV (it may be difficult to place the fiber/catheter)

Box 8.2 Contraindications to endovenous procedures

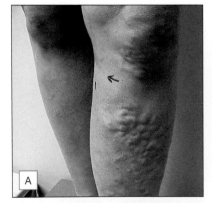 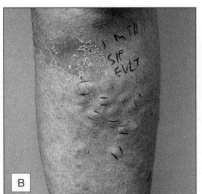 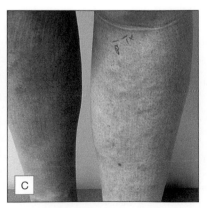

Fig. 8.1 Varicose veins before (**A**), 1 month after endovenous laser of the GSV (**B**), and 1 month after sclerotherapy of residual varices (**C**)

recommends using RFA to treat veins 2–12 mm in diameter, as measured with the patient in the supine position. Some experts use external compression and high-volume tumescent anesthesia to treat veins larger than 12 mm in diameter.

Experienced centers generally report short-term occlusion of the GSV in about 90–95% of patients. Data on file with the company (VNUS Medical Technologies, Inc.) reports that 92% of patients who are reflux-free at 1 year remain so at latest follow up to 5 years (Fig. 8.2).

Randomized prospective studies have found patients treated with RFA experienced shorter postoperative recuperation time, faster return to work and normal activity, and higher quality of life (QOL) scores than patients treated with vein stripping.

Expected Benefits: Endovenous Laser Ablation

The following wavelengths are in current use for EVLA: 810 (DIOMED diode lasers, Diomed Inc., Andover, MA; Ceralas D15/810 diode laser, biolitec, Inc., East Longmeadow, MA), 940 (Dornier D940 Diode Laser System, Dornier MedTech Americas, Inc., Kennesaw, GA), 980 (Ceralas D – 980 nm Diode Laser, biolitec, Inc., East Longmeadow, MA; Precision 980 Vein Laser, AngioDynamics,

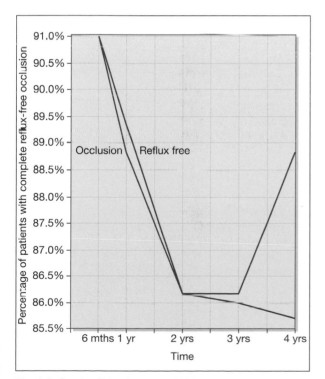

Fig. 8.2 Graph of VNUS Medical Technologies, Inc. data showing percentage of patients with occlusion and reflux-free occlusion

Queensbury, NY), 1064 and 1320 nm (CoolTouch CTEV CoolTouch, Roseville, CA). A study from China found a holmium laser (2078 nm) yielded good short-term success in closing the GSV.

Vein wall injury is probably mediated, regardless of the wavelength used, both by direct effect and indirectly via laser-induced steam generated by heating of small amounts of blood within the vein. The latter mechanism explains the circumferential and homogenous injury found following EVLA, which leads to fibrotic occlusion of the vein. Water is the main chromophore of 1320 and 2078 nm lasers while other wavelengths used for EVLA primarily target hemoglobin. Preliminary reports suggest there may be lower levels of bruising and soreness following EVLA using a 1320 nm laser. But belief in the good short-term efficacy and tolerability of 1320 nm is based on sparse data, with only three patients followed to 1 year and no reports of longer term efficacy. At this time, there appears to be more similarity than difference in results among the various utilized wavelengths. Early data with 810 nm and 940 nm devices suggests treatment failure is very uncommon in patients treated with > 70 J/cm. A withdrawal rate of 2 mm/second at 14 W delivers 70 J/cm.

Short-term success, defined as vein closure on ultrasound at 6–12 months' follow-up, has been reported to be between 90–100%. Min et al found a recurrence rate of < 7% at 2 years in 499 GSVs treated with 810 nm, with no further recurrences in 40 GSVs seen at 3 years. As with RFA, if the vein is closed at 6 months it is unlikely to recanalize. There is level 4 evidence (results from case series) that QOL is better in the postoperative period in those treated with EVLA than in those treated with surgery.

Required Skill Set

The knowledge and skills the physician and treatment team should possess to perform endovenous techniques are listed in Box 8.4.

Overview of Treatment Strategy

Treatment approach

A logical treatment plan can only be constructed after obtaining an appropriate history, and physical examination and diagnostic testing, typically with DUS. The traditional approach to treat GSV incompetence has been surgical ligation and stripping. Alternative treatments for saphenous incompetence include EVLA, RFA and ultrasound-guided sclerotherapy.

Major determinants

EVLA and RFA are less invasive alternatives to ligation and stripping that can be performed in the office setting, under local anesthesia and without incisions. Neovascularization, thought to be a major source of recurrence following ligation and stripping, appears to be much less common following endovenous procedures. This may be because the

---

Skill set required for endovenous techniques

- Knowledge of venous anatomy, disease, physiology and pathophysiology
- Ability to perform a directed history and physical
- Ability to perform DUS for venous diagnosis, mapping, percutaneous access, intraoperative monitoring, and follow-up assessment
- Knowledge of available treatment options, risks, benefits, and contraindications
- Knowledge and technical skill to perform endovenous laser/RF ablation
- Knowledge of proper postoperative care
- Knowledge and skill to perform ancillary procedures, such as sclerotherapy, ultrasound-guided sclerotherapy, and/or ambulatory phlebectomy
- Understanding potential complications and how to prevent, recognize, and manage them

Box 8.4 Skill set required for endovenous techniques

junctional tributary flow is not disturbed. The total cost (cost of the procedure plus societal cost) of endovenous procedures is likely equal to or better than that of surgery. These techniques are being rapidly adopted and probably are being performed more often than traditional stripping in the United States.

EVLA and RFA both appear to be effective treatments for saphenous incompetence. Advantages of EVLA over RFA include shorter procedure times and lower per-treatment cost. Disadvantages of EVLA may include more bruising and discomfort in the early postoperative period. Both techniques continue to undergo refinement, which will likely improve results. Both procedures, when performed using tumescent anesthesia, are associated with low complication rates.

An emerging treatment for saphenous reflux is the use of foamed sclerosants, delivered under ultrasound control. A gas, such as air or CO_2, can be mixed with liquid detergent sclerosants to create foam, estimated to be about four times more potent than the liquid form of the same agent. Early results suggest this may be a valuable modality, as it is quick and inexpensive to perform with reported short- and medium-term success rates of about 80%.

There are many variables regarding foam (e.g. type and amount of gas infused, technique used to create foam, concentration and type of sclerosant used, volume injected, etc.) It is likely that there is a higher risk of deep vein thrombosis (DVT) following foam sclerotherapy. Proper technique is important to minimize the risk of this complication. Other side effects reported following foam include visual and neurological events. To date, there are no reports of long-term visual or neurological complications. Further experience and research with this emerging modality will better delineate its risks as well as long-term efficacy.

Patient Interviews

See Box 8.5 for a checklist of patient information to be obtained.

Treatment Techniques

Patients

Endovenous treatment is indicated in ambulatory patients with incompetence of the GSV who also have associated surface varices, venous symptoms and/or complications of venous disease. Contraindications are listed in Box 8.2.

Equipment

Some equipment and supplies are common to EVLA and RFA, including:

Power table, DUS, sterile gowns, gloves, masks, drapes, gauze, tape measure, ultrasound gel, ultrasound probe and cord cover, antiseptic preparation fluid, local anesthetic, No. 11 blade, 18–19 gauge needle

---

Checklist of information to be obtained from the varicose vein patient

- General medical history
- Current medications/treatments
- If pregnant or breastfeeding
- Medication allergies
- Onset and course of leg veins
- Type of leg veins noted: spider, bulging, abdominal, and pelvic veins
- Symptoms: aching, heaviness, pain, cramping, restless legs, pruritus, leg fatigue, or other symptoms
- Factors exacerbating symptoms: standing, sitting, menses, heat, end of the day, or other symptoms
- Factors improving symptoms: compression stockings, leg elevation, exercise, or other factors
- Complications of venous disease: edema, venous thromboembolism (when, what, how treated), spontaneous hemorrhage, pigmentation, lipodermatosclerosis, venous ulceration
- Current and past vein treatments and outcomes: compression, sclerotherapy (liquid and foam), cutaneous laser, ambulatory phlebectomy, ultrasound-guided sclerotherapy, endovenous procedures, stripping/stab avulsion, anticoagulation
- Diagnostic tests: DUS examinations (when, for what, results)
- Any difficulty with ambulation (physical limitations, travel plans, etc.)
- Family history of spider/varicose veins, ulcer, venous thromboembolism

Box 8.5 Checklist of information to be obtained from the varicose vein patient

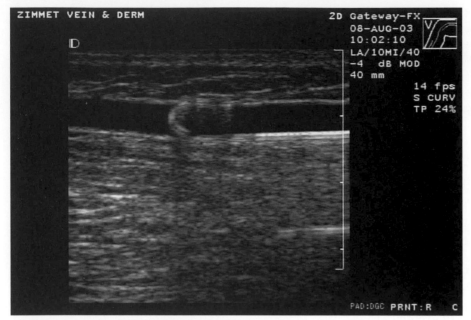

Fig. 8.3 Ultrasound image of J-tipped guidewire in the GSV

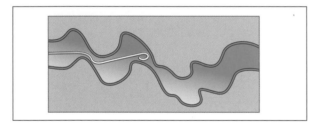

Fig. 8.4 J-tipped guidewire unable to transverse a tortuous vein

for percutaneous entry, 21 gauge spinal needle for administration of tumescent anesthesia, syringes, introducer sheath sets (i.e. sheath, dilator and 0.035 in J-tipped guidewire) and compression stockings and/or bandages. Micropuncture kits are useful when accessing small veins.

Additional materials required to perform EVLA include the laser and sterile laser fiber. Additional components needed for RFA include the VNUS radiofrequency generator, RF catheters (6 Fr or 8 Fr), heparinized saline, and intravenous access set, pole and pressure bag. The 6 Fr catheter expands to 8 mm and the 8 Fr to 12 mm. A 0.025 in guidewire is useful when the catheter fails to advance easily (Figs 8.3 and 8.4).

A rubberized Esmark (Curine Laboratories, Monrovia, CA) or similar bandage may be used intraoperatively. The EVLA and RFA manufacturers preassemble kits containing most of the required supplies.

The cost to purchase a laser ranges from approximately $30,000–70,000, with a disposable cost of about $325 per case. The VNUS RF generator costs less at about $30,000, but disposables are more expensive, costing $825 per case. See Box 8.6 for a cost–benefit analysis.

Tumescent anesthesia

EVLA and RFA should be performed under local anesthesia using large volumes of a dilute solution of Lidocaine and epinephrine (average volume of 200–400 mL of 0.1% Lidocaine with 1:1,000,000 epinephrine) buffered with sodium bicarbonate. This should be delivered either manually or with an infusion pump such that upon completion of the process the vein is surrounded along its entire length with the anesthetic fluid along the segment to be treated (Fig. 8.5).

The benefits of tumescent anesthesia for endovenous techniques are listed in Box 8.7. Although the maximum safe dosage of Lidocaine using tumescent technique for venous procedures is not well studied, a dosage of 35 mg/kg is a reasonable estimate. While tumescent anesthesia in the context of liposuction has been shown to be extraordinarily safe, patients concurrently medicated with other drugs also metabolized via the cytochrome P450 pathway may have slightly

---

Benefit/cost analysis of endovenous procedures done in-office

Cost assumptions

Laser 1	$30,000
Laser 2	$70,000
RF generator	$30,000
EVLA disposables (per case)	$325
RFA disposables (per case)	$825
LVLA facility/staff costs (per case)	$150
RFA facility/staff costs (por case)	$175

Income assumptions

Laser 1	$2041
Laser 2	$2041
RFA	$2216

Benefit/cost ratio (50 cases annually)

Laser 1	3.43
Laser 2	2.70
RFA	1.98

Benefit/cost ratio (100 cases annually)

Laser 1	3.82
Laser 2	3.32
RFA	2.09

The cost of the laser/radiofrequency generator, disposables and facility/staff are estimates. Straight-line depreciation over a 5-year term is assumed for the capital expenditures. The income assumptions use the national average the Centers for Medicare and Medicaid Services have established for EVLA and RFA to treat a single vein. This benefit/cost analysis is from the standpoint of the physician's practice

Box 8.6 Benefit/cost analysis of endovenous procedures done in-office

---

Benefits of tumescent anesthesia in endovenous ablation

- Anesthesia
- Thermal sink, which reduces peak temperatures in perivenous tissues
- Vein compression, which maximizes the effect of treatment on the vein wall

Box 8.7 Benefits of tumescent anesthesia in endovenous ablation

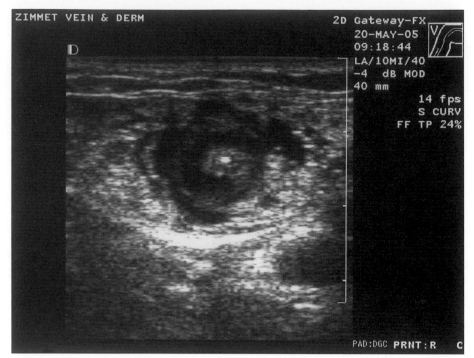

Fig. 8.5 Tumescent anesthetic fluid surrounding the GSV. The sheath/fiber is seen as a bright white image in the center of the photo

slower elimination of Lidocaine, requiring dose adjustment. More information is available at *http://www.liposuction.com/pharmacology/ drug_interact.php*.

Treatment algorithm

The steps common to both EVLA and RFA are:

1. Carry out preoperative assessment, patient education and discussion of risks, benefits and alternatives (informed consent), baseline photographs.
2. Undertake DUS mapping of incompetent underlying venous segments to be treated, including marking of the SFJ and access site (Fig. 8.6).
3. Prepare the operative tray and equipment.
4. Carry out sterile preparation and draping of the leg to be treated.
5. Visualize the access site with DUS.
6. Anesthetize the access site.
7. Insert a 19gauge needle into the GSV under ultrasound guidance. Use a micropuncture set if the GSV is < 4 mm.
8. Place a 0.035 in J-tipped guidewire through the needle into the vein.
9. Confirm the proper placement with ultrasound.
10. Remove the needle and place the introducer sheath with a dilator over the wire. Nick the skin as needed to facilitate entry of the

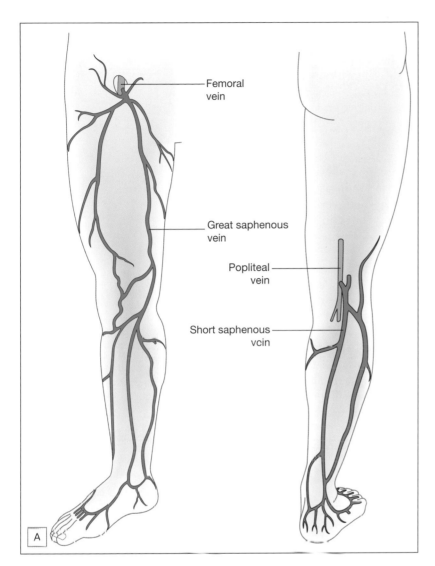

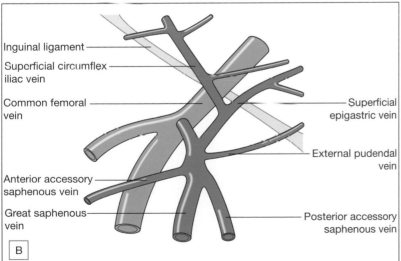

Fig. 8.6 (A) GSV and SSV. **(B)** Anatomy of the right saphenofemoral junction: AL = anterolateral tributary, FV = femoral vein, IL = inguinal ligament, GSV = great saphenous vein, PM = posteromedial tributary, SCI = superficial circumflex iliac vein, SE = superficial epigastric vein, EP = external pudendal vein. Modified from a drawing by Pentti Rautio

sheath through the skin. Confirm intravenous placement with ultrasound.

11. Advance the sheath for RFA its full length (for 6 Fr and 8 Fr, 7 or 11 cm, respectively). Position the sheath in EVLA to about 1 cm below the SFJ.

12. Remove the wire and then the dilator. Check for venous return by aspirating the syringe attached to the sheath.

Additional steps for EVLA include:

1. Place appropriate laser safety goggles on everyone in the operative suite and use other appropriate laser safety measures.

2. Connect the laser fiber to the laser and verify proper laser settings. Setting recommendations vary, but aim to deliver about 70 J/cm length of vein treated: at 14 W this is achieved with a pullback rate of 2 mm/second.

3. Position an appropriately marked laser fiber (manufactured with SiteMarks (EVLT Laser Fiber, Diomed Inc., Andover, MA) or manually mark the laser fiber 3 cm longer than the sheath with a Steristrip) through the sheath so that the tip of the fiber is flush with the tip of the sheath.

4. Withdraw the sheath to the Steristrip/second SiteMark to reveal 3 cm of the proximal laser fiber and then lock the fiber and sheath together.

5. Fine tune the location of the tip of the laser fiber to about 1 cm below the SFJ and below the superficial epigastric vein.

6. Using ultrasound, mark the point at which the vein has been accessed so that treatment can be stopped at that site.

7. Deliver tumescent anesthesia and then place the patient in the Trendelenburg position. Re-verify placement of the laser tip with ultrasound and by viewing the aiming beam through the skin. In addition, the known length of the marked fiber can be used to ascertain tip location (Figs 8.7 and 8.8).

8. Re-verify laser settings.

9. Withdraw the laser fiber and sheath at about 1–2 mm/second with the laser in continuous mode.

10. Stop laser energy delivery at the distal aspect of the vein and place the laser in standby mode.

11. Use DUS to evaluate the treated vein, which should be collapsed.

12. Remove the fiber/sheath from the vein.

13. Record the watts, laser on-time, total joules delivered and length of the segment treated. Calculate the withdrawal rate and joules delivered per cm.

Additional steps for RFA are as follows:

1. Connect the RF catheter to the RF generator.

2. Connect the pressurized heparinized saline drip to the RF catheter.

3. Extend the electrodes into sterile normal saline solution, activate the test button on the generator and check impedance readings. Impedance should be 100–150 Ω (6 Fr) and 40–70 Ω (8 Fr).

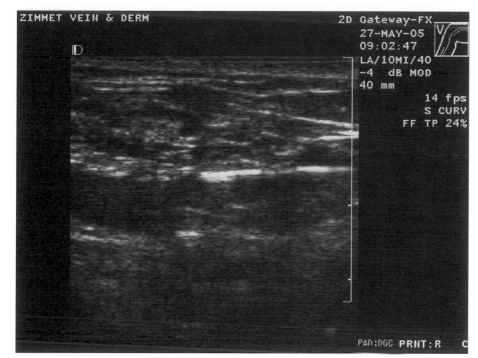

Fig. 8.7 DUS image of laser fiber tip in the GSV below the saphenofemoral junction

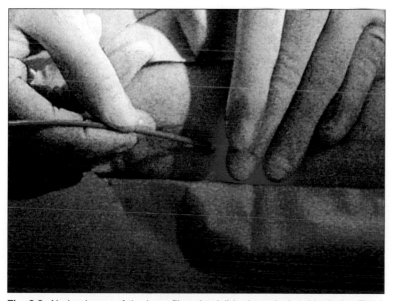

Fig. 8.8 Aiming beam of the laser fiber tip visible through the skin during EVLA

4. Place the RF catheter through the sheath and advance the tip under ultrasound control to just below the SFJ. Use a 0.025 in guidewire if the catheter fails to traverse the vein easily.

5. Check that the heparinized saline is flowing, extend the electrodes, and re-test the catheter. Impedance should be > 200 Ω (6 Fr catheter) or > 150 Ω (8 Fr). Verify that the extended electrodes are 1–2 cm below the SFJ and below the superficial epigastric vein (Fig. 8.9).

6. Deliver tumescent anesthesia and place the patient in the Trendelenburg position.

7. Recheck the position of the extended electrodes.

8. Activate the generator and begin withdrawal of the RF catheter 15 seconds after the target temperature is reached, at about 2.5 cm/minute if using 85°C and about 4.0 cm/minute at 90°C.

9. During withdrawal, keep the vein wall temperature within 3°C of the target temperature while utilizing < 6 W. Impedance should be > 150 Ω (6 Fr) and > 100 Ω (8 Fr). An error message appears in case of excessive temperature or abnormal impedance. Common conditions that cause impedance abnormalities include poor electrode–vein wall contact and coagulum at the thermocouple tip. If impedance is low, increase electrode–vein wall contact by increasing external compression. If impedance is high, coagulum may have formed on the tip. Stop the procedure, adjust the catheter bead such that the length of catheter inserted is marked, remove the catheter, and irrigate any coagulum at the

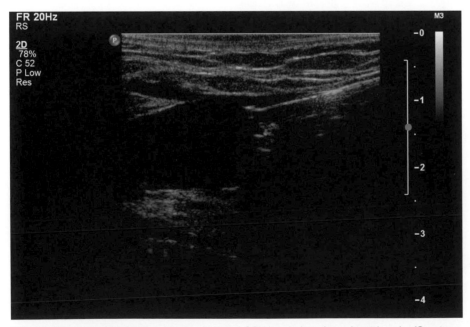

Fig. 8.9 RF electrodes deployed in the proximal GSV just below the epigastric vein. (Courtesy of Dr Nick Morrison)

tip. The catheter can be reinserted to the marker bead, tested, and treatment restarted.

10. Cease treatment when the catheter tip enters the introducer sheath. A sudden increase in impedance signals this has occurred. Remove the RF catheter.
11. Use DUS to evaluate the treated vein, which should be collapsed.
12. Remove the sheath.
13. Record the parameters, duration of treatment, and length of segment treated.

Ancillary treatments, such as ambulatory phlebectomy or sclerotherapy can be performed at the same time as an endovenous procedure (Fig. 8.10).

Postoperative Care and Instructions

Postoperative care is designed to improve efficacy and minimize the risk of complications. Immediately postoperatively, class II compression stockings (30–40 mmHg) are applied and worn for at least 1 week. Short-stretch bandages may be used to reduce bruising and postoperative soreness. They arc applied prior to donning the stocking. Patients should ambulate for at least 20 minutes before leaving the office and at least 1 hour daily for 1 week. Hot baths, heavy lifting and straining should be avoided for 1 week. Nonsteroidal anti-inflammatory drugs may be taken on an as-needed basis for pain. A

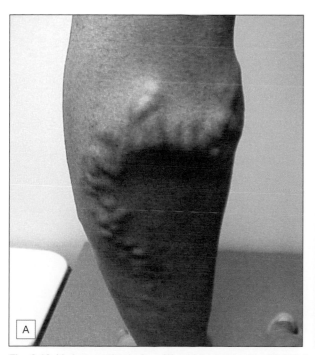
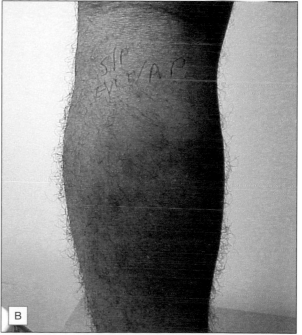

Fig. 8.10 Varicose veins before (**A**) and 1 month after (**B**) EVLA of the GSV and ambulatory phlebectomy of surface varices

follow-up visit and DUS screening for DVT and should be carried out at 3–7 days postoperatively.

Troubleshooting

Percutaneously accessing the vein may be the most challenging aspect of performing endovenous techniques. Several tips can facilitate the successful completion of this key maneuver. The room should be warm and the patient comfortable, in a reverse Trendelenburg position. Anxious patients prone to vasospasm may benefit from oral anxiolytics, such as clonidine (0.1 mg). For sedating and use to reduce anxiety without impairing respiration, clonidine may also safely be given in combination with low-dose lorazepam (1 mg). A micropuncture kit can facilitate accessing small-diameter veins. Striving to place the needle on the first attempt can obviate the need for multiple punctures, which often induce vasospasm. If vasospasm does occur, options include moving proximally for vein access or stopping and waiting for the spasm to subside. In some cases it may be best to stop the procedure, have the patient ambulate for 15 minutes and then try again. A venous cutdown is rarely necessary (Fig. 8.11).

Once a vein has been accessed, rapidly proceeding with insertion of the guidewire and introducer can reduce the risk of vasospasm. If the sheath is in the vein but advancement is difficult, injecting normal saline solution through the sheath may be effective. A 0.025 in guidewire can be placed through the radiofrequency (RF) catheter to aid in placement.

If the tip of the laser fiber or RF electrode is not visible on ultrasound following placement, the tip may be in the common femoral vein or within the introducer sheath. The tip may also be obscured if

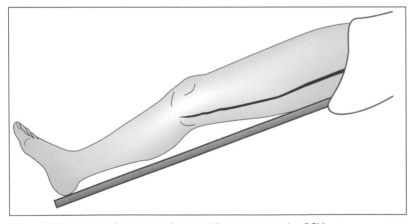

Fig. 8.11 Venous cutdown procedure enabling access to the GSV

the patient is obese. Another way to localize the tip entails visualization of the aiming beam (with laser procedures) followed by measuring the distance from the point of access using the known length of the inserted fiber/catheter.

Side Effects, Complications, and Alternative Approaches

Both EVLA and RFA appear to have a low risk of significant complications. Although bruising and soreness are common after both procedures and may be more significant with EVLA, these effects appear to be mild in most patients and resolve spontaneously. During EVLA, withdrawal of the laser fiber in continuous mode rather than pulse mode can result in reduced bruising and soreness. Reactions to bandages and compression stockings include blisters and dermatitis. Local paresthesias seem to occur in about 1–5% of EVLA patients and about 5–15% of those treated with RFA. Typically resolving over a few months, paresthesias may last longer, with those persisting 1 year reported in about 3% of patients following RFA. Hyperpigmentation, which typically also resolves spontaneously, may occur in about 1% of patients. Skin burns, reported during the early days of RFA, are now rare to nonexistent as long as adequate tumescent anesthesia and proper technique are used. Restricting treatment to veins that are at least 1 cm below the skin reduces the risk of skin burns, paresthesias and pigmentation.

Although a study by Hingorani et al reported a 16% incidence of DVT following RFA, most reports suggest an incidence of about 1%. A small number of DVTs have been reported after EVLA, primarily in patients treated under general anesthesia. Clinical phlebitis can occur after either procedure in about 10% of patients. Infection remains an extremely rare possibility. There is a single report of an arteriovenous fistula that developed following EVLA of the SSV (Fig. 8.6A).

Ultrasound-guided sclerotherapy could be carried out in the event of a localized treatment failure or eventual recanalization. Should RFA or EVLA be completely ineffective, it may be reasonable to consider re-treatment with EVLA/RFA, ultrasound-guided sclerotherapy, or surgical ligation and stripping.

Advanced Topics: Treatment Tips for Experienced Practitioners

Endovenous techniques are used widely to treat the incompetent GSV. Using similar protocols, there are early reports on the use of these techniques to treat other truncal sources of reflux, such as the SSV and anterior accessory GSV. It is important to ensure adequate tumescent fluid around the SSV to protect the sural nerve and to separate the vein being treated from adjacent vessels. When treating the SSV it is prudent to withdraw the laser fiber/RF catheter at a rate quicker than that used to treat the GSV. See Figures 8.12 and 8.13 for before and after photographs.

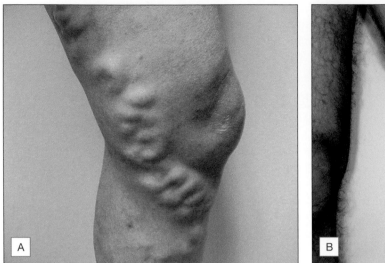 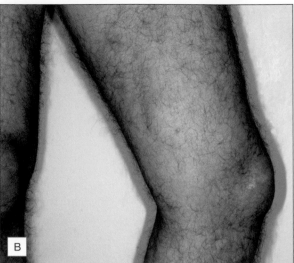

Fig. 8.12 (**A**) 53-year-old white male with symptomatic varicose veins and an incompetent GSV. He underwent endovenous laser ablation with ambulatory phlebectomy of surface varices, followed by 1 sclerotherapy. (**B**) The after photo is 6 months after treatment

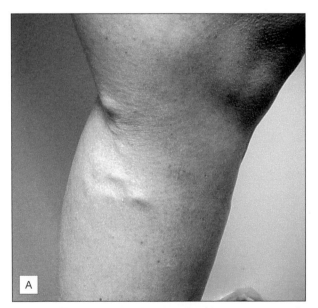 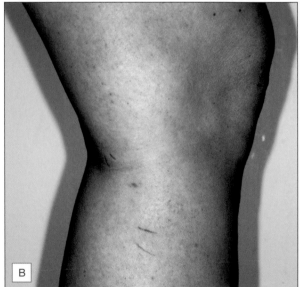

Fig. 8.13 (**A**) 34-year-old white female with very symptomatic varicose veins of the left leg. The EVLT done to incompetent left GSV. (**B**) The GSV was closed on ultrasound at follow up 6 weeks later. The patient stated that her leg feels much better. The mild residual varices will be treated with sclerotherapy

Further reading

Goldman MP, Maritess M, Rao J 2004 Intravascular 1320-nm laser closure of the great saphenous vein: A 6- to 12-month follow-up study. Dermatologic Surgery 30:1380–1385

Hingorani AP, Ascher E, Markevich N, et al 2004 Deep venous thrombosis after radiofrequency ablation of greater saphenous vein: a word of caution. Journal of Vascular Surgery 40:500–504

Lurie F, Creton D, Eklof B, et al 2003 Prospective randomized study of endovenous radiofrequency obliteration (closure procedure) versus ligation and stripping in a selected patient population (EVOLVeS Study). Journal of Vascular Surgery 38:207–214

Merchant RF, DePalma RG, Kabnick LS 2002 Endovascular obliteration of saphenous reflux: a multicenter study. Journal of Vascular Surgery 35:1190–1196

Min RJ, Khilnani N, Zimmet SE 2003 Endovenous laser treatment of saphenous vein reflux: long-term results. Journal of Vascular Interventional Radiology 14:991–996

Min RJ, Zimmet SE, Isaacs MN, Forrestal MD 2001 Endovenous laser treatment of the incompetent greater saphenous vein. Journal of Vascular Interventional Radiology 12:1167–1171

Perkowski P, Ravi R, Gowda RC, Olsen D, Ramaiah V, Rodriguez-Lopez JA, Diethrich EB 2004 Endovenous laser ablation of the saphenous vein for treatment of venous insufficiency and varicose veins: early results from a large single-center experience. Journal of Endovascular Therapy 11:132–138

Proebstle TM, Krummenauer F, Gul D, Knop J 2004 Nonocclusion and early reopening of the great saphenous vein after endovenous laser treatment is fluence dependent. Dermatologic Surgery 30(2 Pt 1):174–178

Proebstle TM, Lehr HA, Kargl A, Espinola-Klein C, Rother W, Bethge S, Knop J 2002 Endovenous treatment of the greater saphenous vein with a 940-nm diode laser: thrombotic occlusion after endoluminal thermal damage by laser-generated steam bubbles. Journal of Vascular Surgery 35:729–736

Rautio T, Ohinmaa A, Perala J, et al 2002 Endovenous obliteration versus conventional stripping operation in the treatment of primary varicose veins: A randomized controlled trial with comparison of costs. Journal of Vascular Surgery 35:958–965

Teruya TH, Ballard JL 2004 New approaches for the treatment of varicose veins. Surgery Clinics of North America 84:1397–1417

Timperman PE 2004 Arteriovenous fistula after endovenous laser treatment of the short saphenous vein. Journal of Vascular Interventional Radiology 15:625–627

Weiss RA, Weiss MA 2002 Controlled radiofrequency endovenous occlusion using a unique radiofrequency catheter under duplex guidance to eliminate saphenous varicose vein reflux: A 2-year follow-up. Dermatologic Surgery 28:38–42

Zikorus AW, Mirizzi MS 2004 Evaluation of setpoint temperature and pullback speed on vein adventitial temperature during endovenous radiofrequency energy delivery in an in-vitro model. Vascular Endovascular Surgery 38:167–174

Zimmet SE, Min RJ 2003 Temperature changes in perivenous tissue during endovenous laser treatment in a swine model. Journal of Vascular Interventional Radiology 14:911–915

Surgical Approaches

9

Joseph R. Schneider, Joseph A. Caprini, with an invited addendum by Andreas Oesch

Introduction

Surgery remains a mainstay of treatment for lower extremity varicosities. Surgery may be as minimal as a local phlebectomy, as discussed in Chapter 7, or as invasive as subfascial endoscopic perforator surgery or stripping of great and small saphenous veins combined with phlebectomy. Surgery must be tailored to the patient's problem. The role of noninvasive testing prior to embarking on surgical correction cannot be overemphasized. This chapter will provide a brief explanation of the major ablative surgical options that may be appropriate in the treatment of patients with lower extremity venous disease. The authors will use the terms 'great' and 'small' to refer to what have previously been termed the 'greater' and 'lesser,' 'long' and 'short,' or 'internal' and 'external' saphenous veins, respectively, following the recent consensus statement on nomenclature.

Stripping of Great and Small Saphenous Veins

Basic concepts, indications and patient selection

Most symptoms in chronic venous disease are due to reflux. For the vast majority of patients treated by experienced clinicians, duplex scanning has replaced all other forms of venous testing, including qualitative assessment of reflux. Patients are tested in the standing position on the upper step of a two-step platform by asking them to stand normally but relaxed on both legs. The great saphenous vein (GSV) is imaged with the patient facing the technologist and the study leg slightly forward and externally rotated.

The vein is examined for dilation, compressibility, and echogenicity in the transverse orientation. The longitudinal view is also assessed, and thickness of the vein wall, valvular changes or any echogenicity is documented (Figs 9.1–9.5). The operator tests for reflux in the axial vein and perforating veins using color flow, and also uses the pulsed Doppler with the probe in longitudinal orientation to test for reflux in the saphenofemoral junction, the common femoral vein above and below the saphenofemoral junction, and the proximal GSV. The Valsalva maneuver is appropriate for provoking reflux in the groin, but may not provoke reflux inferior to the groin if there is a competent

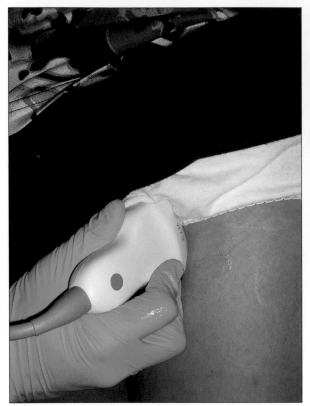

Fig. 9.1 Linear array duplex probe in longitudinal orientation about to be applied to upper anteromedial left thigh/groin to interrogate the underlying femoral vein and saphenofemoral junction with color flow and pulsed Doppler

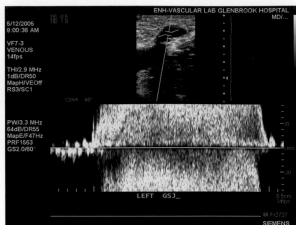

Fig. 9.2 Duplex scan image and Doppler spectrum from interrogation of the saphenofemoral junction with pulsed Doppler using the probe position as in Figure 9.1. The patient's head (superior) is left and foot (inferior) is to the right on the image in the upper portion of the frame. The lower portion of the frame is the Doppler blood flow signal over time coursing from left to right. Flow demonstrated above the 0 line on the spectrum represents reflux during the Valsalva maneuver. In this case, there is gross reflux with 'aliasing' of the Doppler spectrum beginning with Valsalva at the first large time tick mark in the lower left part of the figure and lasting longer than 2 seconds

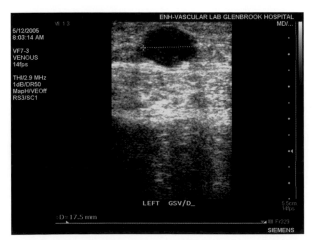

Fig. 9.3 Transverse image of the GSV in the mid-medial thigh. The vein is the relatively echolucent (dark) oval in the upper center portion of the frame. The vein is patent and dilated (17.5 mm)

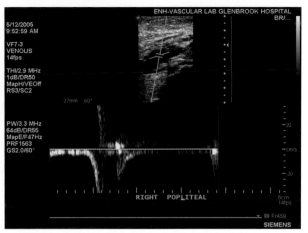

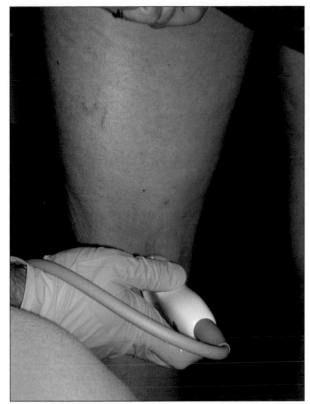

Fig. 9.5 Duplex scan image and Doppler spectrum from interrogation of the popliteal vein just superior to the saphenopopliteal junction with pulsed Doppler using the probe position as in Figure 9.4. The patient's head (superior) is left and foot (inferior) is to the right. In this case, there is prograde flow with compression of the calf (Doppler detected flow below the 0 line and 'aliasing' above the 0 line just after the first large time tick mark in the lower left portion of the frame) and no reflux is demonstrated (no sustained significant flow above the 0 line) with release of calf compression

Fig. 9.4 Linear array duplex probe in longitudinal orientation applied to the left popliteal region (posterior) to interrogate the underlying popliteal vein and saphenopopliteal junction with color flow and pulsed Doppler

valve in the groin area. Therefore, compression of the leg above and below the segment being interrogated is used to detect evidence of reflux in the target segment. For example, saphenofemoral and proximal great saphenous reflux may be masked during the Valsalva maneuver by the presence of a competent valve in the proximal common femoral vein. The author tests for this by squeezing the upper thigh between two hands (lateral and medial) while interrogating the proximal GSV with pulsed Doppler and looking for 'to and fro' flow. The Valsalva maneuver may also fail to demonstrate reflux in the more inferior segment of the GSV and the practitioner must depend on proximal and distal compression maneuvers to elicit reflux when it is significantly inferior to the saphenofemoral junction.

The small saphenous vein (SSV) is examined for dilation and reflux with the patient standing and facing away from the technologist and the popliteal vein is imaged from this approach as well. Examination of the SSV is started at the ankle posterior to the lateral malleolus. The course of the vein is traced proximally where it very quickly drifts to the midline of the calf and can clearly be identified within its superficial fascial compartment. Branches and connections are usually seen in the mid-calf and the operator eventually traces these branches but not until the entire course of the SSV is studied.

The examination is done in the transverse view until the whole course of the vein is mapped. Often the vein will extend proximally past the popliteal fossa and sometimes eventually connects to the GSV in the groin as the so-called vein of Giacomini. The SSV is also interrogated in the longitudinal view near the popliteal fossa to document the saphenopopliteal junction. This is a critical step since the SSV may empty into a gastrocnemius branch, which then enters the popliteal fossa. If this is not well understood and observed by the surgeon, important errors can occur and precipitate damage and/or thrombosis of the deep venous system.

Careful documentation is required of reflux, valve anatomy and any vessel defects in the common femoral and popliteal veins, with the operator specifically looking for evidence of previously unsuspected deep venous abnormalities, which if present dictate a conventional supine venous duplex scan of the entire deep venous system. Evidence of significant chronic abnormalities in the deep vein system would not necessarily preclude any planned ablation of the superficial veins but further consideration and discussion with the patient may be necessary.

Correction of superficial venous insufficiency in the presence of deep venous insufficiency may improve the patient's clinical degree of disability but does not obviate the necessity of wearing appropriate heavy compression stockings. This must be carefully explained to the patient since many patients assume that surgery will render obsolete the wearing of these hose. Stockings are the best treatment and prophylaxis for deep venous insufficiency, and long-term compliance is the key to success, especially postoperatively.

Being physically present to conduct the exam with the technologist is important to the surgeon's understanding of the patient's pathophysiology and to the eventual success of any contemplated operation. Readers interested in a more detailed description of diagnostic standards may wish to consult Mattos and Sumner or Nicolaides.

Stripping procedures

The first description of 'stripping' of the GSV is generally credited to Babcock. This operation is most commonly considered for patients with primary varicose veins, usually clusters of varicose branches of the GSV adjacent to (and probably communicating with) the various named perforating veins connecting the deep and superficial veins of the medial leg. The strategy of this approach is to ablate the major axial conduit through which venous hypertension is transmitted from the level of the right atrium to the superficial veins of the leg in patients with venous valvular incompetence. Furthermore, ablation of the axial vein theoretically leads to thrombotic occlusion of any perforating veins that communicate directly with the GSV. However, the effectiveness of stripping for perforator ablation is less certain, especially below the knee, where the major axially directed vein that connects with the Cockett perforating veins is the posterior arch (Leonardo) vein, which is not ablated by a conventional stripping operation (Fig. 9.6).

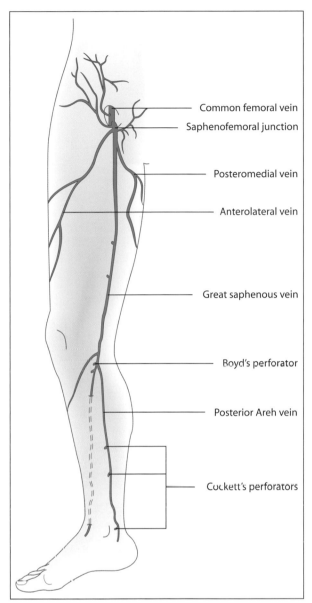

Common femoral vein

Saphenofemoral junction

Posteromedial vein

Anterolateral vein

Great saphenous vein

Boyd's perforator

Posterior Areh vein

Cockett's perforators

Fig. 9.6 The important perforating veins below the knee communicate with the posterior arch vein (Leonardo), not the axial GSV

The ideal patient for classic stripping of the GSV will have: (1) a dilated GSV (> 8 mm in diameter adjacent to the saphenofemoral junction) with saphenofemoral or proximal great saphenous reflux lasting at least 1.5 seconds; (2) clusters of varicose branches in the thigh; (3) absence of significant perforating vein reflux; and (4) no evidence of significant changes of deep vein thrombosis (DVT). Removal may still be indicated in certain patients with distal communicating branches off a normal-caliber GSV with reflux, or with dilatation of the GSV without observable reflux. In practice, most patients have areas of the GSV much larger than 8 mm in diameter and reflux lasting much longer than 1.5 seconds. The location of the lowest connecting perforator, which is often in the distal thigh or very proximal calf, is marked during the duplex examination since removal of the vein below this level is unnecessary and increases the chance of saphenous nerve injury (Fig. 9.7).

Small saphenous vein (SSV) stripping is performed less often and when it is performed, it may be limited to a segment and not the entire SSV. The superior termination of the SSV is variable (Fig. 9.8) and must be clearly delineated at the time of any diagnostic imaging study to provide sufficient information on which therapeutic decisions may be based. It may be useful to re-image the patient just before surgery and to mark the location of the SSV and its termination at and above the knee to allow accurate placement of incisions. This may even be performed in the operating room with the patient prone on the

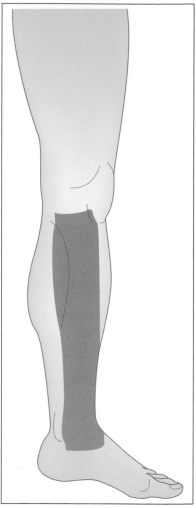

Fig. 9.7 The saphenous nerve is adjacent to the GSV and at most risk of injury from the upper calf to the ankle

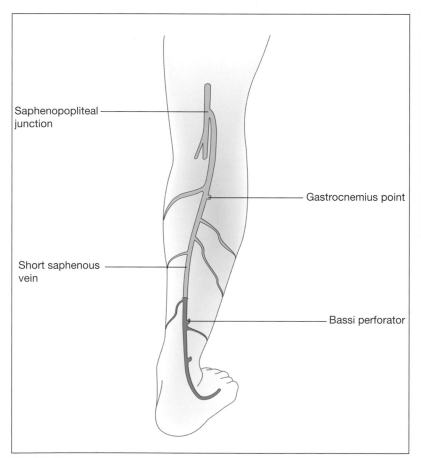

Fig. 9.8 The most common communication between the SSV and the deep vein system is a direct communication with the popliteal vein within 5 cm of the popliteal crease. However, up to one-third of patients may have a termination more than 5 cm away (usually above) the popliteal crease and 10% or more will have no communication in the posterior thigh and the vein will continue superiorly as a vein of Giacomini

operating table. SSV segments at least 4 mm in diameter with demonstrable reflux can be considered for stripping. It is rarely necessary to remove the distal third of this vein, and normally the vein can be removed to the proximal or mid-calf just below the last major communicating varicosity identified during the duplex examination.

Technique

Subarachnoid block (spinal) or general anesthesia is used when classic stripping operations are performed. In the majority of patients, the GSV may be removed using two small incisions. One incision in the groin crease just medial to the femoral pulse usually allows easy exposure of the proximal GSV and saphenofemoral junction (Fig. 9.9).

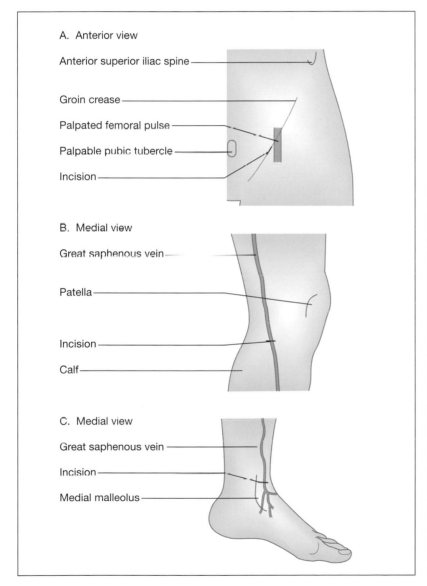

A. Anterior view

Anterior superior iliac spine

Groin crease

Palpated femoral pulse

Palpable pubic tubercle

Incision

B. Medial view

Great saphenous vein

Patella

Incision

Calf

C. Medial view

Great saphenous vein

Incision

Medial malleolus

Fig. 9.9 Typical incisions used for classic stripping of the great saphenous vein. The left leg is illustrated. (**A**) An approximately 3 cm incision is placed in the groin crease just medial to the femoral pulse. This incision usually provides excellent exposure of the saphenofemoral junction, but should be extended as needed, especially in obese patients to allow adequate safe exposure and secure identification of the branches. (**B**) The great saphenous vein becomes relatively superficial in the uppermost calf and a 2.5 cm incision in the upper posteromedial calf usually allows identification and control of the GSV to allow stripping of the thigh segment of the GSV. (**C**) In cases where it is felt necessary to remove the GSV in the calf, the vein is usually easily identified and controlled with a 2.5 cm incision at the superior anterior aspect of the medial malleolus. A transverse incision tends to be longer, but tends to heal with a less prominent scar than does a longitudinally oriented incision at the ankle. The practitioner must be careful to separate the GSV from the saphenous nerve to avoid injury of the latter when exposing the vein at the ankle

The incision should be large enough to provide adequate exposure to allow a complete and safe procedure, particularly in obese patients. The incision should not be made inferior to the groin crease since an inappropriately inferior incision would make control of branches other than the GSV more difficult.

It is appropriate to obtain control of the GSV, but to not ligate the vein at this point for reasons that will become apparent later. First, the operator may attempt to identify all other branches, most often including the anterolateral saphenous, external pudendal, superficial epigastric, and circumflex iliac branches (Fig. 9.10). Each of these latter branches is then divided and attempts made to ligate each of their primary branches as well to reduce the risk of persistent or recurrent communication between the deep and superficial venous systems in the groin. The posteromedial aspect of the common femoral vein is inspected, with frequent attendant identification and division of a small (2–4 mm) branch in this area that might contribute to recurrences. At the completion of this portion of the operation, the axial GSV is the only remaining unligated branch at the saphenofemoral junction.

The authors have noted that it was necessary to remove only part of the GSV in a majority of more than 1500 patients. In many such cases, the vein may be removed from knee to groin using a second incision placed medially at the level of the knee instead of at the medial malleolus. Use of the retrograde pin-stripping technique as described by Oesch (*vide infra*) may allow even more limited surgical trauma to the patient, but still allow adequate removal of abnormal axial GSV (Fig. 9.11). The key is appropriate preoperative documentation by duplex scan of the venous anatomy. In many patients, dilatation, reflux, and incompetent perforators will end at or just below the knee.

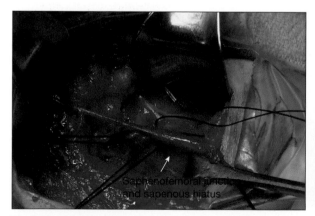

Fig. 9.10 Extensive dissection of the saphenofemoral junction. The patient's head is to the left and feet are to the right. It is important to ligate the tributaries of the saphenofemoral junction including the anterolateral, superficial epigastric, external pudendal, and circumflex iliac branches as well as the primary branches of these veins in addition to the axial great saphenous vein to reduce the risk of neovascularization and recurrence

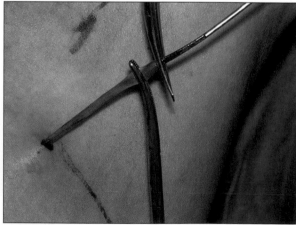

Fig. 9.11 Use of the pin stripper to remove a segment of the GSV. The pin stripper has been passed retrograde from the left saphenofemoral junction and brought out though a small stab wound in the medial thigh. The pin stripper is pulled out through the stab wound and the vein is everted during removal

There is no need to remove any more of the normal vein without incompetent associated perforators and this more limited approach reduces the risk of saphenous nerve injury. Failure of the surgeon to be present at the diagnostic duplex scan venous evaluation makes this essential operative decision difficult to make. When the entire GSV is dilated with reflux, it is necessary to remove the axial GSV. The vein can be identified through an incision at the medial malleolus. By dissecting carefully on the top of the vein and carefully cleaning it posteriorly, the risk of saphenous nerve injury can be minimized.

When using the classic technique, the operator may ligate the vein in the inferior aspect of the knee or at an ankle level incision, inserting the end of the disposable plastic Codman stripper wire (Arrow Medical, Libertyville, IL) through a venotomy superior to the point of ligation. The stripper wire is then advanced superiorly through the GSV up to the groin, where it almost always appears in the vein identified as the GSV. This allows an independent confirmation that the proper structures have been identified in the groin.

Occasionally the stripper is observed to appear in the femoral vein in the groin, implying that the wire has entered the deep venous system, presumably through a perforator somewhere in the leg. Obviously, this would mandate removal of the wire and repeat passage until the wire appeared where expected. It is theoretically possible for the stripper wire to enter the deep system through a perforator and then return to the GSV through another perforator, although the authors are not aware that this has ever been documented. Some surgeons prefer passing the wire from the groin toward the ankle, but many prefer to be reassured that the wire appears where expected in the groin when passed from ankle to groin. It is thought that passing the stripper from a distal position to a proximal one and stripping from a proximal to a distal one may reduce the chance of injury to the saphenous nerve.

The stripper wire is next brought out of the vein through a venotomy in the superior portion of the GSV and the vein is ligated around the stripper wire and divided at the ankle or knee. The saphenofemoral junction is divided, ligated and suture ligated proximally flush with the femoral vein. The Codman handle is placed on the inferior (ankle or knee) end of the stripper wire and the small or medium Codman 'stripper head' is attached to the superior end of the wire (Fig. 9.12). The stripper is pulled from groin to knee and allowed to exit at the knee incision in the case when only the superior half of the vein is to be removed.

An umbilical tape is tied to the wire just inferior to the stripper head in cases when the entire vein (ankle to groin) is to be removed. The vein is then partially stripped by pulling the stripper down to the mid-calf area. The handle is rapidly removed and replaced with the small Codman stripper head at the inferior end of the stripper wire. The umbilical tape is used to pull the wire back into the groin, thus allowing upward stripping of the distal end of the vein with a smaller head, with a hoped for reduction in the risk of injury to the saphenous nerve. Some prefer to use reusable Fischer metal wire strippers

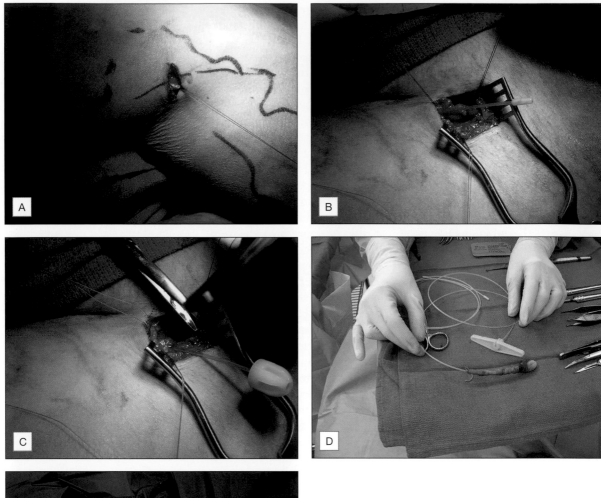

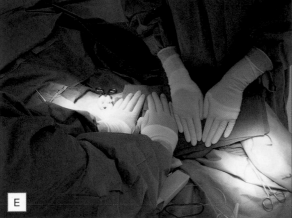

Fig. 9.12 (**A**) The left GSV has been controlled at the level of the knee anticipating passage of the Codman stripper from the knee to the groin. The black lines indicate the varicose branches marked prior to surgery to be removed using the stab phlebectomy technique. The purple line is the predicted course of the great saphenous vein before the incision is made. (**B**) The Codman stripper has been passed from the knee to the groin, seen here from the patient's left side. (**C**) The medium stripper head has been placed on the superior end preparing for downward stripping of the thigh segment of the great saphenous vein. (**D**) The vein has been stripped from the groin to the knee and is seen reefed onto the Codman stripper. (**E**) Pressure is held over the course of the vein that has been stripped

(VENOSAN North America, Asheboro, NC) that have either no head or much smaller heads than the Codman stripper. Particularly when removing a major portion of the GSV, this device helps minimize surgical trauma to the leg. An epinephrine-soaked gauze roll may be packed into the thigh portion of the bed of the GSV and the leg may also be elevated at this point. Both of these maneuvers are designed to reduce bleeding into the tract of the vein from avulsed side branches and perforating veins. In all cases, pressure is held over the bed of the vein for a measured 7 minutes. In some cases it may be preferable to operate with the legs elevated on a foot bracket to minimize bleeding, with subsequent wrapping of the thigh with a 6 in elastic bandage for at least 10 minutes following removal of the GSV. In this manner, ablation of the GSV is completed.

Oesch has also described a method he has termed 'pin-stripping.' Rigid metal strippers (also VENOSAN North America) are thus used to remove segments of vein up to 50 mm in length. Pin-stripping is generally performed by passing the wire in a superior to inferior (retrograde) fashion along the path of reflux. Significantly, inadvertent passage of the pin stripper into the deep system through a perforator is nearly impossible. Pin-stripping may be used as a first-line technique and is also an excellent alternative in cases where the conventional stripper wire cannot be passed in a distal to proximal direction. The approach may be accomplished with strictly local anesthesia coupled with a standard groin incision and dissection for the GSV and its branches.

While the pin stripper is usually passed retrograde from the groin down to the distal point of reflux determined by preoperative duplex scanning, it is equally effective when passed in a distal to proximal direction. In the latter case, the process can be repeated to remove additional portions of the vein, usually starting at the ankle where the superficial course of the vein can be palpated. Whether passed proximally or distally, the 'leading' end of the pin stripper may then be passed through the vein wall and up to the skin under which it may be felt and through which it may be brought out through a small puncture wound. Any questionable area should be left untreated until post-operative duplex-guided techniques can be used to complete the vein removal without damage to the deep venous system (see Figs 9.11 and 9.13).

The pin-stripping method is associated with a very low rate of recurrence at the groin. Furthermore in those patients with recurrences who have returned for duplex evaluation, no cases of neovascularization have been observed following these techniques. Pin-stripping appears to be particularly useful for incompetent and varicose anterolateral branches reached via the retrograde approach from the groin (Fig. 9.14).

Rivlin is most often credited with development of a technique to treat the SSV, which is best approached with the patient in the prone position. As noted earlier, the variability in how the SSV communicates with the deep venous system mandates careful duplex imaging.

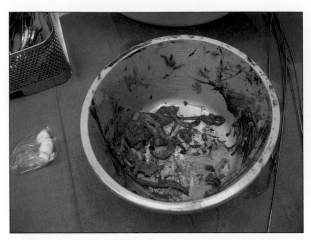

Fig. 9.13 Example of retrieved volume of varicosities after combined ankle-to-groin stripping and stab phlebectomy. The large and medium Codman stripper heads are seen within the small plastic bag to the left of the basin. The metal pin strippers are seen to the right of the basin

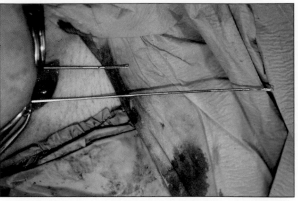

Fig. 9.14 Parallel stripping of the great saphenous and anterolateral branch. The pin strippers have been passed retrograde from the right saphenofemoral junction into both veins to be brought out through stab wounds in the thigh

Identification of reflux in the superior end of the SSV requires that the vein be ligated superiorly at a point where the practitioner can be certain there are no branches between the point of ligation and the communication with the deep venous system. This often requires a transverse incision at or above the popliteal flexion crease, allowing the surgeon to follow the small saphenous vein to its junction with the popliteal vein, taking great care not to injure other structures in the popliteal fossa, such as the popliteal vein, artery and tibial nerve. The sural nerve is adjacent to the SSV essentially throughout the latter's course in the lower leg and care must be taken not to injure this nerve during surgery. The SSV is almost always removed using a pin stripper. Removal of the SSV using the pin stripper takes advantage of the 'invagination' technique, which may produce less tissue trauma, may be less likely to injure the sural nerve, and is particularly advantageous when only the superior end of the vein is abnormal and only a portion of the vein is to be removed (Fig. 9.11). The pin stripper is advanced distally until the last major perforator in the SSV is passed. The pin stripper can then be brought out through a puncture wound in the skin and after ligating the proximal end of the vein and attaching it to the pin stripper. The vein can be removed in a proximal to distal direction by invagination. Note, as previously stated, that removal of the distal SSV is seldom required.

Results

Stripping of the GSV with concomitant phlebectomy is an effective and durable procedure for primary varicose veins. Dwerryhouse and colleagues reported three of 52 (6%) of their patients required reoperation at 5 years after a conventional knee-to-groin stripping operation. This compared with 11 of 58 (19%) patients who had undergone ligation at the saphenofemoral junction alone. Both of these groups underwent concomitant local treatment of the associated varicose tributaries. Despite the observation that 29% of patients undergoing knee-to-groin stripping had a duplex scan demonstrating reflux in the residual (infragenicular) GSV, the results of this investigation imply that these patients did very well without ablative treatment. A follow-up investigation yielded life-table estimates of freedom from re-operation at 11 years to be 86% after stripping.

Use of Phlebectomy vs. Sclerotherapy as an Adjunct to Stripping of Axial Veins

The majority of patients with symptomatic superficial venous hypertension will have significant branch varicosities. Bergan has argued that these are related by location and pathophysiology to named perforating veins, particularly in the distal thigh and upper calf. One way to treat these branches is to perform sclerotherapy once the underlying hemodynamic problem has been addressed by stripping of the axial vein. However, while sclerotherapy may provide good early results with minimal discomfort, experience has shown that phlebectomy, as covered in Chapter 7, is probably more effective and durable in the longer term. Furthermore, it is more efficient to combine both the stripping and treatment of branch varicosities in one procedure (Fig. 9.13). Branch varicosities will have been marked with the patient standing using indelible marker either in the office on the day before surgery or in the holding area just prior to surgery (Fig. 9.15).

Muller is often credited with the earliest modern description of the technique of local phlebectomy, which may have been used as long as 2000 years ago. During the past 40 years, development of specialized

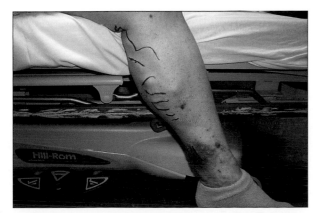

Fig. 9.15 Varicose branches to be removed in surgery should be marked with permanent marker with the patient standing in the office or in the holding area prior to surgery, since they will be much less apparent when the patient is recumbent on the operating table

hooks has allowed local phlebectomy through ever smaller wounds. Most practitioners use a technique similar to that described by Muller and modified by Oesch, Ramelet and others. When Oesch hooks are used, they may be inserted through small wounds created with a No. 11 scalpel or 18 gauge needle. Some authors have argued that phlebectomy should be performed before stripping of the axial vein because of the extreme venous hypertension that occurs at the time of stripping. Finally, the transilluminated powered phlebectomy shows promise as a new technique to achieve complete removal of branch varicosities.

Removal of Infragenicular Great Saphenous Vein

The saphenous nerve accompanies the GSV from just below the knee to beyond the medial malleolus and is at risk during surgery on the infragenicular portion of the vein. Thus, some have argued that the vein should only be stripped from the knee to the groin using a small incision in the posterior medial knee area for access. Some have even argued that the direction in which the stripper is pulled is important. However, not all authors agree that the risk of injury to the saphenous nerve is altered by limiting stripping to the knee-to-groin segment of the GSV. Furthermore, the late sequelae of saphenous nerve injury, while common, may be of little or no practical consequence.

Finally, the residual infragenicular GSV has been found to be significantly abnormal (refluxing) in a substantial fraction of patients in whom it has been preserved by stripping only from knee to groin. The grossly dilated proximal GSV may be most appropriately treated with a medium-sized stripper head, but the authors are reluctant to pass this in either direction along the segment from the mid-calf to the ankle because its bulk may injure the adjacent saphenous nerve in the confined subcutaneous space typically found in the lower leg. Instead, the small stripper head may be used. Postoperative persistent, symptomatic saphenous neuropathy is rare after ankle-to-groin stripping of the GSV. Alternatives include use of the Oesch invagination technique or the metal stripper with a very small head.

Simple Ligation of Saphenofemoral Junction

Trendelenburg is thought to have been the first to advocate ligation of the saphenofemoral junction to reduce ambulatory venous pressure in the superficial veins inferior to the saphenofemoral junction. This procedure has been advocated by some as a method to preserve the axial GSV for possible use as an arterial bypass conduit. Others have used this minimally invasive approach to alleviate the venous hypertension and allow more durable treatment of branch varicosities, either by phlebectomy or sclerotherapy. However, this approach is relatively likely to fail; in contradistinction, the likelihood of recurrence is reduced if, at the same time, the knee-to-groin segment of the GSV is stripped in association with treatment of branch varicosities.

Subfascial Endoscopic Perforator Surgery (SEPS)

Basic concepts, indications and patient selection

Conservative treatment of venous ulcers with elevation and compression is associated with a significant rate of failure to heal and frequent recurrence even in highly compliant patients. This was noted as early as 1867 by Gay as cited by Rhodes and Gloviczki. Linton recognized the contribution of perforating veins to superficial venous hypertension and developed a radical operation to ligate perforating veins and thereby isolate the deep and superficial venous systems. However, Linton's operation was associated with a substantial risk of wound complications (approximately 25%) and less than certain healing of venous ulcers. Modification of the Linton procedure by others resulted in some reduction in complications, but wound problems were still present in an unacceptable fraction of treated patients. This morbidity appears to be related in part to the creation of large flaps with concomitant compromise of skin perfusion. Hauer appears to have been the first to report a less invasive endoscopic approach for interruption of incompetent perforating veins, with Bergan the first to use the term 'subfascial endoscopic perforator vein surgery' (SEPS) in the English language.

The basic premise in perforator interruption is that ulcers relate to persistent ambulatory venous hypertension and that incompetent perforating veins contribute to ambulatory venous hypertension. Indeed, ulceration is rare with isolated superficial venous incompetence, and hemodynamic studies of patients with venous ulcers have shown that 73% have incompetent calf perforating veins combined with either superficial or deep venous reflux. Thus, stripping of the great saphenous vein alone is unlikely to be effective in healing venous stasis ulcers.

Patient selection for SEPS

Surgeons continue to explore the appropriate indications and role of SEPS in patients with venous stasis ulcers. The ideal patient to consider for this therapy has a classic medial supramalleolar venous stasis ulcer, hemodynamic evidence of incompetent perforating veins, and no evidence of deep venous thrombosis. The procedure, like the original Linton procedure, was initially reserved for patients with advanced stasis dermatitis and open ulcers (CEAP class 6), but early encouraging results have led many surgeons to extend the procedure to patients in CEAP Class 5 or even Class 4. Noninvasive testing, again dominated by duplex scanning, is the primary method of patient testing when the practitioner is considering SEPS, and such testing is critical for preoperative mapping of incompetent perforating veins. Normal perforating veins are difficult or impossible to identify with duplex scanning, but incompetent perforating veins are generally easily identified by the presence of dilation and reflux. The leg is scanned with the same basic technique as is used for varicose vein studies by sweeping a linear probe in transverse orientation along the medial side of the leg. It is important to be certain that the patient has no evidence of deep vein thrombosis (DVT), acute or chronic, as DVT may significantly and negatively impact the efficacy of SEPS. Perforating veins are identified and checked for reflux using color flow and pulsed Doppler interrogation (Fig. 9.16) and are marked with indelible marker on the surface of the skin to allow later interruption during SEPS. In order to obtain the best results, duplex scanning and mapping should be overseen by both the surgeon and ultrasound technologist.

Technique

SEPS has generally been performed with either general or regional (subarachnoid block or epidural) anesthesia, but it may be possible to perform SEPS with tumescent anesthesia. The perforating veins that are the target of this surgery may be located anywhere between the medial posterior edge of the tibia and the posterior mid-line of the calf. It is this subfascial area that must be dissected to make the perforating veins available for interruption. Most important medial perforating veins communicate with the posterior arch vein, but there is some communication with the axial GSV near the knee.

While access to the subfascial space of the lower leg is usually obtained through incisions in the upper or mid-medial calf, the technique is performed with some variation from center to center. For example, Hauer used a single port and Pierik has described a technique using a single port with a mediastinoscope. The Loma Linda group (Bianchi) uses a single port technique as well. The Mayo Clinic Group has described the procedure performed with two ports (one for a laparoscopy scope and the other for working) (Fig. 9.17), an

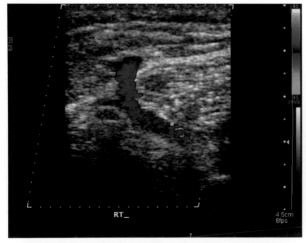

Fig. 9.16 Reflux is demonstrated in this large perforating vein during the Valsalva maneuver

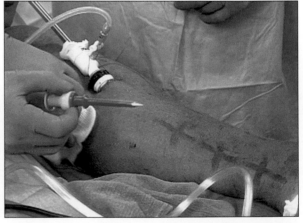

Fig. 9.17 Left leg SEPS using a two-port system. Three large incompetent perforators have been marked prior to surgery using the duplex scanner. The camera port and camera are already in place. The working port in the surgeon's right hand is about to be placed inferior and posterior to the camera port. (Courtesy of Roy Tawes MD)

exsanguinated limb, a pneumatic tourniquet on the thigh, and the use of CO_2 insufflation used to perform much of the dissection. Conrad has described a similar procedure with CO_2 insufflation, but without exsanguination and tourniquet. The more recent two-port approaches are very attractive because smaller wounds are required and visualization is improved because a capacious working space can be maintained with CO_2 insufflation. However, a CO_2 insufflation maintained working space is now possible with the single port approach as well. A commercial system has also become available that uses two ports, does not require exsanguination, and uses balloons to complete much of the dissection (United States Surgical, Norwalk, CT).

Whichever technique is used, the perforating veins must be identified and interrupted using clips (Fig. 9.18), a harmonic scalpel, or another technique. Anatomic considerations may dictate entry into the deep posterior compartment and are considered by some to be mandatory to ensure that all perforating veins have been addressed. The very distal Cockett I perforating veins may not be reachable with the endoscope and associated tools, and may require a separate incision in the area of the medial malleolus. SEPS is often combined with ablation of the GSV or other appropriate procedures designed to deal with superficial venous reflux. Indeed, this is viewed as critical to the success of SEPS when the patient has concomitant great saphenous incompetence.

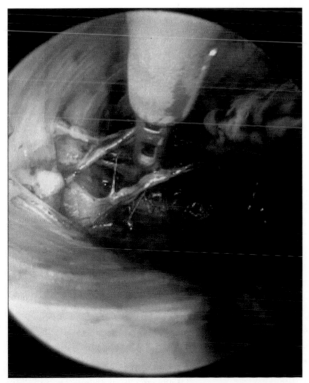

Fig. 9.18 Endoscopic view of perforators being clipped during SEPS. (Courtesy of Roy Tawes MD)

Results

Pierik et al published the results of a randomized study comparing SEPS to a conventional open perforator interruption (Linton operation) for venous ulcers. These authors noted no wound complication after SEPS vs. a 53% rate of major wound complications after open perforator ablation, and they noted no recurrence of ulceration in either group. There was no nonsurgical treatment arm in their study. Even so, with the single exception of the Pierik study, there are to the authors' knowledge no prospective randomized trials of SEPS vs. alternative therapies for ambulatory venous hypertension with ulceration. Despite the absence of Level I evidence, early short- and medium-term results are quite encouraging with respect to morbidity, early ulcer healing, and freedom from recurrent ulceration.

Rhodes and Gloviczki have provided a tabulation of the available and evaluable early series of SEPS. The series are diverse. Some of these articles are inexplicit with respect to preoperative clinical status (CEAP classification) and hemodynamic status (testing). Many operations include ablation of the GSV, and follow up is often short or indeterminate. Nevertheless, it is useful to note that of well over 400 limbs treated with SEPS, only about 5% suffered wound complications, 90% enjoyed initial healing of ulcers, and only 12% were observed to have recurrent ulcers. The latter observation must be qualified by saying that follow up was often short or indeterminate, but the aggregate of these studies gives reason for optimism that SEPS will provide successful healing and prevention of ulcers in a clear majority of patients with a low risk of complications. Tawes et al recently described the results of SEPS in 832 patients using a single protocol for evaluation and treatment in five different centers. They reported only 8% failed to heal their ulcer or experienced '...no benefit from the operation...' and only 4% suffered recurrent ulceration or other deterioration from 6 months to 2 years after SEPS. TenBrook et al reviewed English language reports of SEPS and found an 88% rate of initial ulcer healing with a 13% recurrence rate by 21 months. However, they also detected a worrisome 7% aggregate rate of neuralgia after SEPS.

The results of open perforator ablation appear dramatically different when comparing patients with primary valvular incompetence to those with post-thrombotic venous hypertension (in a post-phlebitic limb). The rate of recurrent ulcers is roughly double in post-thrombotic limbs compared to primary valvular incompetence limbs (46% vs. 20% estimated recurrence rate at 2 years using life-table comparisons). Interestingly, this seems to parallel the observation that hemodynamic improvement is more likely after SEPS in primary valvular incompetence than in postphlebitic limbs. The reader is cautioned to take these observations into account when making therapeutic decisions and counseling potential SEPS candidates. However, it appears that up to two-thirds of patients with venous stasis ulcers suffer from primary venous valvular insufficiency and not 'postphlebitic syndrome' and, thus, at a minimum, should be considered candidates for SEPS or direct deep venous valvular surgery.

Summary

Particularly in the context of large and complex varicosities, stripping of the great and small saphenous veins remains an essential part of the treatment of superficial venous incompetence. Techniques have evolved that minimize complications, including injury of the saphenous and sural nerves. SEPS is an emerging technique that holds promise for alleviating venous hypertension and healing stasis ulcers in highly selected patients.

Addendum by Andreas Oesch, Bern

Indications for Surgery Today

Phlebectomy

Endovenous treatments of varicose veins by laser or radiofrequency heat application are increasingly promoted, suggesting that the heyday of venous surgery is over now. However, few are the cases where these nonsurgical treatments alone will suffice. If saphenous insufficiency is such that treatment is clearly indicated, varicose side-branches will need additional phlebectomy or sclerotherapy. As the leg is already anesthetized, the logical option is phlebectomy, which in this situation is also safer and more reliable than injection therapy. When saphenectomy is performed following the pin-stripping method, the GSV or SSV is selectively removed to the distal point of incompetence. Most varices start from this point and are pulled out together with the saphenous vein, which permits an easy and integral resection of the complete reflux pathway.

Extended varices

To reduce the evident risk of skin burns, endovenous heat treatments should be performed under tumescent anesthesia. This elegant and well-tolerated anesthesia has two drawbacks: it is rather time consuming and it is limited in its application. If the required volumes of anesthetizing solution would reach critical levels in patients presenting extended varices, two treatment sessions are advisable. In these cases, leave of absence from work and costs will exceed the ones caused by a single surgical treatment.

Small saphenous vein

Any treatment of the SSV can induce lesions of the sural nerve, which – in contrast to the less insidious saphenous nerve – tend to be persistent and painful. Selective stripping of the incompetent segment of the SSV is associated with a high risk of thermal injury to the closely adjacent sural nerve. Anesthesia for pin-stripping of the SSV requires only limited infiltration restricted to the junction and the tributaries, and takes very little time!

Short proximal reflux

In this situation, only a short part of the saphenous vein needs to be inactivated, e.g. from the groin to mid-thigh or from the popliteal to mid-calf. The crossectomy incision is used for inserting the stripper. The vein segment is easily removed by pin-stripping, even in obese patients. On the other hand, distal introduction of a probe starting at the terminal point of saphenous reflux is difficult. The usual approach is to insert the probes for thermal ablation at the ankle or below the knee, thus sacrificing a good portion of healthy vein.

Complex anatomical patterns

Varices in the thigh are frequently perfused both by the anterolateral vein and the GSV itself. The two reflux systems should be eliminated. As they are separated by just a few centimeters of tissue, this step is only permitted when performed in an atraumatic way. The crossectomy permits open resection of the complex junction (which usually includes an aneurysmal dilatation of the beginning of the anterolateral vein) and pin-stripping of both veins. This 'double-stripping' also reveals the varicose connections between the two reflux systems.

Complex reflux patterns switching between the GSV stem and large parallel tributaries are rather common. Obliteration of all pathways without touching intact segments by endovenous procedures (or sclerotherapy) is difficult or even impossible in obese patients. Classic Babcock stripping removes the complete stem notwithstanding its variable pathophysiology and leaves the refluent tributaries in situ. Pin-stripping permits surgically following the reflux network by re-introducing the probe at the points where the flow is deviated.

Special localizations

Perforators in critical areas such as the knee joint cannot be treated safely by thermal procedures. Surgery in local anesthesia helps to avoid neurological complications. The only alternative is ultrasound-guided sclerotherapy.

The deep-lying Giacomini vein with its small diameter is difficult to treat. In my opinion, the best method is pin-stripping from the popliteal junction to the GSV. Care has to be taken to avoid deviating the probe into the deep venous system.

Lack of competency in endovenous procedures

Early reports on the radiofrequency treatment show complications by far exceeding those of stripping procedures. Most of them are minor problems, such as skin burns, sensory loss and indurations, but there is also an alarming incidence of DVT involving the femoral vein. Increasing experience seems to reduce the complication rate to the level of surgery, albeit proximal DVT is apparently an inherent problem of thermal occlusions. Precise placement of the probe below the junction with correct temperature adjustment is probably the clue to reduce DVT without compromising good long-term results. For endovenous treatments, sound practical knowledge of ultrasound techniques is mandatory. Unfortunately, endovenous devices are often propagated as easy methods for everyone to perform, where technology may be a substitute for practical skills and experience.

Limited financial resources

Endovenous laser and radiofrequency treatment are high-tech procedures. Generators as well as nonreusable probes are expensive and high-quality imaging systems required. When financial resources are scarce, the application of these techniques is simply impossible. In patients with a high income, the initial expenses may be counterbalanced by a shorter time off work.

Conclusion

Surgery still has its place in the treatment of venous disease. The propagators of new technologies often overemphasize the negative aspects of stripping by comparing the newcomers with outdated surgical methods. Actual surgery means selective stripping by invagination and hook phlebectomy. This minimally invasive approach has low rates of thrombosis, few sensory losses and almost no skin problems, and compares very favorably with any other therapeutic option. The cosmetic results are good and there is little postoperative pain. Nevertheless, GSV stripping has two disadvantages: unpleasant bruising of the thigh and varicose recurrence in the groin. Bruising can be reduced by immediate local compression of torn tributaries. In my patients, an inverting suture of the femoral stump has proved to be effective against inguinal revascularization.

The epidemiology of vein diseases has changed within the last decades. Today patients present with milder forms of varices; in the same time these patients have become more demanding. Consequently less invasive treatment concepts for treating the simpler forms of varicose veins have been developed. It is not clear if these are suited for extensive and complex situations or if they will stand the test of time. At the present time surgery is still the first choice for complicated forms of varicose veins.

Further reading

Aremu MA, Mahendran B, Butcher W, et al 2004 Prospective randomized controlled trial: conventional versus powered phlebectomy. Journal of Vascular Surgery 39:88–94

Bergan JJ 2001 Surgical management of primary and recurrent varicose veins. In: Gloviczki P, Yao JST (eds) Handbook of Venous Disorders. 2nd ed. Arnold, London, pp 289–302

Bergan JJ 2002 Varicose veins: hooks, clamps, and suction. Application of new techniques to enhance varicose vein surgery. Seminars in Vascular Surgery 15:21–26

Bergan JJ, Murray J, Greason K 1996 Subfascial endoscopic perforator vein surgery: a preliminary report. Annals of Vascular Surgery 10:211–219

Bianchi C, Ballard JL, Abou-Zamzam AM, Teruya TH 2003 Subfascial endoscopic perforator vein surgery combined with saphenous vein ablation: results and critical analysis [see comment]. Journal of Vascular Surgery 38:67–71

Caggiati A, Bergan JJ, Gloviczki P, Jantet G, Wendell-Smith CP, Partsch H 2002 Nomenclature of the veins of the lower limbs: an international interdisciplinary consensus statement. Journal of Vascular Surgery 36:416–422

Conrad P 1994 Endoscopic exploration of the subfascial space of the lower leg with perforator vein interruption using laparoscopic equipment: a preliminary report. Phlebology 9:154–157

Conrad P, Gassner P 1996 Invagination stripping of the long and short saphenous vein using the PIN stripper. Australia and New Zealand Journal of Surgery 66:394–396

Dwerryhouse S, Davies B, Harradine K, Earnshaw JJ 1999 Stripping the long saphenous vein reduces the rate of reoperation for recurrent varicose veins: five-year results of a randomized trial. J Vasc Surg 29:589–592

Fronek A, Denenberg JO, Criqui MH, Langer RD 2003 Quantified duplex augmentation in healthy subjects and patients with venous disease: San Diego population study. Journal of Vascular Surgery 37:1054–1058

Gloviczki P, Bergan JJ, Rhodes JM, Canton LG, Harmsen S, Ilstrup DM 1999 Mid-term results of endoscopic perforator vein interruption for chronic venous insufficiency: lessons learned from the North American subfascial endoscopic perforator surgery registry. The North American Study Group. Journal of Vascular Surgery 29:489–502

Hauer G 1985 Die endoskopische subfasziale Diszision der Perforansvenen: vorläufige Mitteilung [Endoscopic subfascial division of perforating veins-preliminary report] Vasa 14:59–61

Kalra M, Gloviczki P 2003 Surgical treatment of venous ulcers: role of subfascial endoscopic perforator vein ligation. Surgical Clinics of North America 83:671–705

Kistner RL, Eklof B, Masuda EM 1996 Diagnosis of chronic venous disease of the lower extremities: the CEAP classification. Mayo Clinic Proceedings 71:338–345

Kistner RL, Eklof B 2001 Classification and diagnostic evaluation of chronic venous disease. In: Gloviczki P, Yao JS (eds) Handbook of Venous Disorders. 2nd edn. Arnold, London, pp 94–103

Labropoulos N, Leon M, Geroulakos G, Volteas N, Chan P, Nicolaides AN 1995 Venous hemodynamic abnormalities in patients with leg ulceration. American Journal of Surgery 169:572–574

Labropoulos N, Mansour MA, Kang SS, Gloviczki P, Baker WH 1999 New insights into perforator vein incompetence. European Journal of Vascular and Endovascular Surgery 18:228–234

Linton RR The communicating veins of the lower leg and the operative technic for their ligation. Ann Surg 107:582–593

Magnusson M, Kalebo P, Lukes P, Sivertsson R, Risberg B 1995 Colour Doppler ultrasound in diagnosing venous insufficiency. A comparison to descending phlebography. European Journal of Vascular and Endovascular Surgery 9:437–443

Mattos MA, Sumner DS 2001 Direct noninvasive tests (duplex scan) for the evaluation of chronic venous obstruction and valvular incompetence. In: Gloviczki P, Yao JST (eds) Handbook of venous disorders. 2nd edn. Arnold, London, pp 120–131

McMullin GM, Coleridge Smith PD, Scurr JH 1991 Objective assessment of high ligation without stripping the long saphenous vein. British Journal of Surgery 78:1139–1142

Morrison C, Dalsing MC 2003 Signs and symptoms of saphenous nerve injury after greater saphenous vein stripping: prevalence, severity, and relevance for modern practice. Journal of Vascular Surgery 38:886–890

Nicolaides AN 2000 Investigation of chronic venous insufficiency: A consensus statement. Circulation 102:E126–E163

Oesch A 1993 'Pin-stripping': A novel method of atraumatic stripping. Phlebology 8:171–173

Pierik EG, van Urk H, Hop WC, Wittens CH 2001 Endoscopic versus open subfascial division of incompetent perforating veins in the treatment of venous leg ulceration: a randomized trial. J Vasc Surg 26:1049–1054

Proebstle TM, Bethge S, Barnstedt S, Kargl A, Knop J, Sattler G 2002 Subfascial endoscopic perforator surgery with tumescent local anesthesia. Dermatologic Surgery 28:689–693

Rhodes JM, Gloviczki P 2001 Subfascial endoscopic perforating vein surgery. In: Gloviczki P, Yao JST (eds) Handbook of venous disorders. 2nd edn. Arnold, London pp 391–400

Ricci S, Georgiev M, Goldman MP 1995 Ambulatory phlebectomy. A practical guide for treating varicose veins. Mosby-Year Book, St Louis

Rigby KA, Palfreyman SJ, Beverley C, Michaels JA 2004 Surgery versus sclerotherapy for the treatment of varicose veins. Cochrane Database of Systematic Reviews CD004980

Stonebridge PA, Chalmers N, Beggs I, Bradbury AW, Ruckley CV 1995 Recurrent varicose veins: a varicographic analysis leading to a new practical classification. British Journal of Surgery 82:60–62

Tawes RL, Barron ML, Coello AA, Joyce DH, Kolvenbach R 2003 Optimal therapy for advanced chronic venous insufficiency. Journal of Vascular Surgery 37:545–551

TenBrook JA Jr, Iafrati MD, O'Donnell TF Jr, et al 2004 Systematic review of outcomes after surgical management of venous disease incorporating subfascial endoscopic perforator surgery. Journal of Vascular Surgery 39:583–589

Index